Contents

Dedication	page iii
Forward	Page iv
Neurodegeneration, a multi-pronged approach	Page 1
Vitamin D	Page 17
Vitamin E	Page 25
Vitamin A	Page 26
Cholesterol	Page 27
Good Fats, Bad Fats	Page 39
Choline	Page 43
Vitamin B complex	Page 47
Vitamin C	Page 53
MND, Exercise and Glutamic Acid	Page 54
Butter not Margarine	Page 64
Alpha Lipoic Acid	Page 68
Salicylates	Page 71
Nicotine	Page 74
High Fat Diets	Page 75
The Problem with Medication	Page 77
Antioxidants, juicers	Page 85
Recipes	Page 92

All rights reserved. No part of this publication may be reproduced, stored in a retrieval system or transmitted in any form or by any means, without prior permission in writing of the author Lynne D M Noble, or as expressly agreed by law, or under terms agreed with the appropriate reprographics right organisation.

You must not circulate this book in any other binding or cover and you must impose the same condition on any acquirer.

Independently published 2018

This book is dedicated to

Joy and Colin Bray

Thanks for your friendship

May every blessing be yours

Forward

On 22/04/18, I attended a talk on MND given by a researcher in this field. The talk included information about the presence of microglia in the brains of those with motor neurone disease. Microglia are the cells found in the brain which mop up inflammation and diseased cells and an excess of microglia appear to be the 'wind fanning the flames' in the progression of MND. Thus, undue numbers of microglia, signal a rapidly advancing pathological process.

Regulatory T cells (Tregs) - which modulate the immune system and prevent auto immune diseases - have been found to decrease during disease progression in Amyotrophic Lateral Sclerosis (ALS)[1] - the most common form of MND. However, when upregulation of Tregs occurred, the progression of activated microglia slowed.

There are a great many fascinating processes going on in the immune system but it is not my intention to discuss them here in any great detail. It is sufficient to say that a number of dietary substances do upregulate Tregs and, as such, have the potential to slow down the rate of progression of motor neuron disease. It is thus the dietary considerations which will form the main foci of this book. However, it is not my intention to discuss how the diet should be implemented. Those with MND will be at different stages of the disease process and some may have problems with swallowing. People have different food

---

[1] https://www.sciencedaily.com/releases/2018/03/180322103318.htm

preferences. Therefore, any specific food may be cooked and presented to meet the need of any individual at any time.

It is not enough for an individual to say that they follow along the lines of 'healthy eating' since healthy eating is not a one size fits all concept. There are diets which are specifically designed to respond to the vagaries of particular illnesses, such as diabetes and iron deficiency anaemia, and MND is no different in that respect. This diet has been carefully researched to respond to current scientific research. This has shown that an increase in Tregs has the potential to slow down the disease process.

The nutritional building blocks required for good brain health are also discussed in this book. It stands to reason that, if nutritional substances which support brain health are not present, then the potential for repair is diminished - where repair is possible. Many antioxidants and nutrients have been well researched and found to slow down neuronal loss. Little of this valuable information appears to have found its way into the literature advising those with MND and their families on healthy eating. For example, coffee – whether caffeinated or decaffeinated – has been found to slow down the rate of progress of MND. This information does not appear to have found its way into literature for patients with MND.[2]

Of course, we all lose some neurons every day and this is accelerated by narrowing of the blood vessels to the brain. According to research, neurons in the central nervous system –

---

[2] https://academic.oup.com/aje/article/174/9/1002/168671

unlike those in the peripheral nervous system - once lost, don't *spontaneously* regenerate. This was thought to be primarily due to inhibitory factors such as chondroitin sulphate proteoglycan which are not present in the peripheral nervous system. However, studies show that the application of the enzyme chondroitinase supports the regeneration of corticospinal lesions in spinal cord lesions.[3]

In addition, numerous other studies have shown that CNS remyelination within the brain and spinal cord can be extensive.[4] The phenomenon of extensive remyelination, which is often see in multiple sclerosis, is one such example. As such, central nervous system axons are capable of regeneration in an appropriate environment.

The destruction of a nerve nucleus is a different matter. The genetic material of the cell is contained within the nucleus. It is where replication occurs and when this is completed, two identical DNA molecules exist. One is the original and the second is the newly created complementary strand.

---

[3] K K Jain MD (Dr. Jain is a consultant in neurology and has no relevant financial relationships to disclose.)
Originally released July 28, 2000; last updated July 10, 2018; expires July 10, 2021

[4] https://academic.oup.com/qjmed/article/107/5/335/1564446

The destruction of the nerve nucleus will result in the muscle atrophy which is commonly seen in MND. Therefore, it is important that undesirable events which potentiate the loss of the nerve nucleus are addressed as soon as possible.

According to studies[5] which have looked at the incidence and mortality rate of motor neuron disease since the 1950's - the rate at which this occurs continues to rise. This may well be due to factors such as increased life expectancy - since MND is more likely to appear in older populations - or better diagnosis of the disease. However, the possibility that the increase of MND is associated with environmental factors – leaning heavily towards nutritional status - cannot be taken out of the equation. To do so would be foolishness. Our diets have undergone rapid and marked changes since the 1950's. When a thorough examination of these changes is made, it appears our 'healthy' lifestyles are not as healthy as we are led to believe. I will explore this in much greater detail in this book as well as how our current lifestyle and beliefs can potentially increase our risk for a neurodegenerative disorder. However, there was a further marked increase in ALS in the 1990's and this coincided with the time when statins were heavily marketed. This will also be explored in line with current research.

Our diets are very different now to those enjoyed in post war Britain. Eggs and butter were eaten freely then. Offal was served up frequently. These foods are anti-inflammatory. Margarine has replaced butter and polyunsaturated vegetable

---

[5] https://www.alzforum.org/news/research-news/lou-gehrigs-disease-rise

oils – erroneously promoted as being healthy - has replaced the lard and dripping once used widely. Polyunsaturated vegetable oil and margarine are both pro inflammatory. Inflammation is the primary root cause of most chronic diseases. It is no wonder that neurodegenerative diseases have risen steadily since the early 1950's. Healthy fats have been replaced by pro inflammatory man-made hydrogenated fats and oils. These are woven into most ready to eat foods found in the supermarkets nowadays.

Saturated fat and cholesterol have been demonised and yet are essential for health. I shall explore this in some detail in this book.

A diagnosis of MND is made when medics have eliminated all other known neurodegenerative diseases. This is unsatisfactory in many respects. The remaining individuals are informed that there is no cure found yet (as though there can only be one specific cause for the condition which afflicts the remaining individuals) for which a treatment may eventually be found. The reality is that, for each individual who has received a diagnosis of MND, it may be a multi-step process involving six diverse steps of, as yet unknown origin.[6] Nevertheless, the out of control microglia point firmly to the underlying aetiology being auto-immune in origin – it has its roots in inflammation which is attacking self. This is something that we can begin to address through diet.

---

[6] The six stage multi step theory is the one currently proposed to model the progression of stages which will ultimately result in the signs and symptoms of MND

Although evidence suggests that ALS may be a multistep - process, there must also be an underlying genetic susceptibility to MND. This means that as well as the contribution of a number of sequential steps leading to a diagnosis of MND there must initially be a genetic susceptibility to the disease. Nevertheless, this should not daunt us from exploring potential causes and responses since genes can be influenced by environmental factors which have the potential to turn genes on and off.

Diet is a major environmental factor which, under this umbrella term, encompasses within it many other nutritional sub domains which may influence the onset of the development of MND as well as other neurodegenerative disorders. Within the concept of 'diet' there are many factors which can predispose to neurodegeneration – either directly or indirectly. It is quite possible that the genetic propensity to MND is played out entirely through the individual's nutritional status.

Correct nutrition – which provides the building blocks of our brain for repair and growth - also detoxifies and provides energy. However, one missing vitamin, mineral or other essential nutrient may mean that a metabolic pathway is hampered with a subsequent impairment or loss of function. An analogy is that when making concrete, my husband tells me we need cement, sand, water and aggregate. If one of the constituents is missing, then it simply is not up to the job; the structure would be weak and eventually collapse.

This analogy demonstrates what might happen if we don't ingest a diet which contains all the necessary nutrients for good health, yet our current lifestyles do not support good neurological health. Our diets have become 'low fat', 'no fat' and low cholesterol, although good fats are necessary for brain health. Our brain contains 60% of fat and approximately 25% of our brains are formed from cholesterol. Some fats cause neuro-inflammation. It is therefore important that the difference between fats which support neurological health and those that don't are understood.

Cholesterol is an essential component of brain tissue but unfortunately has also been demonised. This substance is essential for many functions in the body, including a healthy brain. Cholesterol will be discussed in detail in this book.

I will give a little space to factors which appear to increase the likelihood of getting MND and the potential reasons for this.

My intentions in writing this book are:

1. To inform. This will include understanding what a bespoke diet which promotes brain health consists of.
2. To identify foods which are known to upregulate T cells which has been found to slow the progression of the disease.
3. To present this material in an easily read and easily understood form, bearing in mind that this book is for those with MND and their families. As such, I will not be including any 'heavy' research in the book although the information in this book is research based. Such a book may well come later but it is not for now.

4. To give a brief introduction to some medications which may actually predispose an individual to MND and other neurodegenerative diseases.
5. To provide tasty and nutritious recipes which promote brain health as well as inspire readers to use food as a medicine. There is a section at the back of this book devoted to this.
6. To learn a little about the antioxidants which promote good brain health and which help to prevent further neurodegeneration.

Why Neurodegeneration Needs a Multi-Pronged understanding and Response.

Neuroscience is a fascinating subject but probably not for the thousands of people who are diagnosed with a neuro-degenerative disorder every year. Some neuro-degenerative disorders can be treated with medications which slow down the process of the disease. However, their effectiveness has been shown to be short lived. The effectiveness of others is in doubt. It is questionable whether any prescribed medication actually prolongs the quality or quantity of life any more than if the medication had not been prescribed.

The four disciplines which offer most to the understanding and treatment of inflammation – the root cause of chronic disease are:-

- **Neuroscience**
- **Immunology**
- **Nutrition**
- **Pharmacology**

The first two disciplines help us to understand the underlying pathological processes contributing to the disease. The second two disciplines help us to provide a response to our understanding of what the aetiology of the medical condition is.

Nutrition is by far the 'Cinderella' of the disciplines and yet bespoke nutrition carries with it a genuine and effective response to neuro-inflammatory conditions. I do not know of anyone yet, suffering with a neuro-degenerative disorder, who has been immediately referred to a dietician or nutritionist so that it can be ascertained whether the individual's diet lacks nutrients essential for neuro health. This is a much neglected area. Suitable dietary responses – as well as many other non-dietary responses - are lacking for neuro-degenerative disorders. It is not clear why.

Conditions such as diabetes and iron deficiency anaemia seem to be understood and addressed well by those working in the field of nutrition. Copious leaflets are produced which are updated as science advances. There have been numerous advances in our understanding of how nutritional status affects neuro health but I have seen precious little finding its way into material which is available for patients. We may not have total understanding of MND but surely we can impart of what we do know that is helpful.

The lack of suitable dietary responses is not something to be proud of for this is often the space that pharmacology fills. There are of course wonder drugs but alongside these there are many noxious substances with severe side effects. These drugs may be prescribed for years before the damaging side effects can be ignored no longer. They will then be taken off the market for causing far worse problems than the symptoms that they were originally designed to treat. You do not have to think hard before Thalidomide and Vioxx (Cox-2 inhibitor) come to mind as examples of this. However, there are many other drugs that have permanently damaged the health of thousands of individuals – often in the pursuit of profit. Some of these – such as statins - are still in use even though they are associated with ALS and type 2 diabetes.

Alan E Nourse[7]

The apothecaries of the middle Ages and Renaissance viewed the human body as an experimental laboratory in which almost any substance could be tested in the hope of finding cures for almost everything. In a very real sense, their customers were the guinea pigs of the day, and often failed to survive the treatment.

This truism is just as relevant today as it was then.

Statins are often (incorrectly) associated with preventing heart disease and are prescribed widely. I will expand on this in more detail in this book. I will also include the potentially negative effects that statins have on the brain as well as general health. Current research shows a link between the prescribing of statins and Type 2 diabetes. This systemic condition impacts on the brain. What we think we know – common knowledge - regarding statins, saturated fat and cholesterol is not born out by many robust studies including the well- known Framingham Heart Study.

There are a number of issues which we need to address when responding to neurodegeneration. These are:

---
[7]

https://trove.nla.gov.au/version/45753613

1. Address neuro-inflammation through regulation of effector T cells and administration of antioxidants (the domains of immunology, and nutrition)
2. Slow down the potential for neuronal/axonal loss (domain of nutrition and possibly pharmacology)
3. Repair or potentiate growth of neuronal fibres (domain of nutrition)
4. Provide structural building blocks for the brain (domain of nutrition)

It can be seen that nutrition is able to respond to all four areas. This shows the importance of what this particular discipline has to offer. Some medications such as steroids do address inflammatory issues but they do have some serious side effects which are better to be avoided if at all possible. In any case steroids are not for long term use. They can cause more damage than they alleviate. However, EPA targets the same inflammatory pathway as steroids do but without the side effects.

Ibuprofen and Indomethacin have far less damaging side effects and have been found to promote axonal regeneration in the central nervous system.[8] As our goal is to promote axonal regeneration where damage has occurred then providing the side effects which can occur through the use of NSAID's – are recognised and managed – then I see no reason why these NSAIDS cannot be prescribed for neuro-inflammatory disorders. An alternative to the above is to introduce more

---

[8] https://www.ncbi.nlm.nih.gov/pubmed/17428993

foods containing salicylates which have an anti-inflammatory action. This will be explored later in the main body of the book.

A further strength of responding to neuro-inflammation by using nutrition as a medicine, is that it is something that everyone can be involved in. It is not a hugely difficult subject to understand since you don't necessarily need to understand the underlying chemistry for it to work – that has already been researched and produced in this book. All you need is the willingness and ability to accommodate a diet which is specifically tailored to respond to the needs of the brain, following the principles set out in this book. However, many people do want to delve further into the fascinating world of nutrition so, to this end, I have added some more in depth information, along the way, for those who want to look into this further.

Vitamin D – the Immune System 'Regulator' which is necessary for brain health

Vitamin D is essential for the overall health of the body. Vitamin D receptors can be found throughout the body and there is marked intracellular distribution of vitamin D receptors in the brain. Developmental vitamin D deficiency has been found to cause abnormal brain development. [9]

Studies[10] have shown an association between low vitamin D levels and a shorter survival time in patients with ALS. Further studies have shown that there was a slower decline in ALS progression scores when patients were treated with 2000 IU's of cholecalciferol daily compared to the control group.

Most people are aware that vitamin D is necessary to build strong bones but it has many other important roles to play in health including a regulatory role in the immune system. This regulatory role – important in auto immune conditions – also impacts on rampant microglia which play such an important part in the progression of MND.

In spite of its importance, it is practically impossible to take in enough vitamin D through diet alone since it is found in only a

---

[9] https://www.ncbi.nlm.nih.gov/pubmed/19500914
[10] Vitamin D confers protection to motor neurons and is a prognostic factor of amyotrophic lateral sclerosis.

Camu W, Tremblier B, Plassot C, Alphandery S, Salsac C, Pageot N, Juntas-Morales R, Scamps F, Daures JP, Raoul C
Neurobiol Aging. 2014 May; 35(5):1198-205.

few foods. Many of these foods do not form a regular part of many people's diet. Further, as we grow older we become less efficient at absorbing most nutrients in our diet and as appetite lessens with age we take in fewer nutrients. These factors all contribute to vitamin D deficiency.

Vitamin D requires fat to aid its absorption, yet our current propensity to very low fat – or no fat - diets hinders this.

Fortunately, this vitamin is also made through the action of sunlight on the skin. The easiest way to get Vitamin D is to expose your skin to sunlight. Your skin does not need to burn in order for vitamin D to be produced. Nevertheless, the amount which can be made in this way depends on:

- the colour of your skin
- how much skin is exposed
- the intensity of the sun's ultraviolet B rays.
- The amount of cholesterol you have since it is the action of the sun's rays on the cholesterol under the skin which helps synthesise vitamin D.

The current fashion of covering up and slapping sun cream on as soon as the sun appears could be causing more harm than good in many respects. I can understand that our pale skins would need some protection if exposed to prolonged intense sunshine such as that found in some countries where the sun's rays are much stronger than to be found in ours. However, most of the time we live in an environment where the sun's rays are quite weak and we do not want to inhibit our capacity to make vitamin D.

Most people understand that vitamin D is necessary for strong healthy bones but they may not be aware that

- vitamin D synthesises an antimicrobial peptide called cathelicidin or
- that it has an essential regulatory function in the brain and body by helping to prevent auto immunity.

among many other vital functions.

Cathelicidin is important, it is part of the innate[11] immune system. Cathelicidin related antimicrobial peptides (CAMP) are key compounds of the innate immune system. They have a broad spectrum anti-microbial action again gram+ and gram- bacteria, viruses and fungi. They have immune modulatory functions including roles in wound healing, the induction of cytokines and altering gene expression.[12] They are produced by many different cells including neutrophils, epithelial cells and macrophages.[13] The presence of vitamin D during macrophage differentiation bestows the capacity to mount an antimicrobial response to kill intra cellular microbes.

Studies have shown that when this anti-microbial peptide is deficient then it was associated with a more marked pro-inflammatory response.[14] Cramp deficient mice displayed a

---

[11] The innate immune system is the one you are born with and responds generally, and not specifically, to infective agents
[12] https://www.ncbi.nlm.nih.gov/pubmed/28082134
[13] Neutrophils and macrophages are cells of the immune system.
[14] https://www.ncbi.nlm.nih.gov/pubmed/23969854

higher degree of glial cell activation that was accompanied by a more pronounced pro-inflammatory responses.

Exposure to the sun for thirty minutes, at least twice a week, should produce adequate amounts of vitamin D for our needs in the summer. However, getting enough vitamin D naturally through the winter time is far more problematical. It is at this time that supplementation with this vitamin needs to be considered for optimum health.

The Recommended Dietary Allowance (RDA) for Vitamin D was originally set at 400 International Units (IU's) in the 1950's. This decision was based on the minimum amount required to prevent rickets – that was all. It cannot adequately sustain a healthy body nor maintain optimum neurological health. There is a huge difference between 'just preventing' illness and 'optimising' overall health.

The current recommendations for vitamin D are between 1,000 and 4,000 IU's. The best form to take is Vitamin D3 which is the active form. Blood tests can easily identify whether you have too little or too much of this vitamin so anyone who has a neurodegenerative disorder should ask for a blood test, from their GP, to establish vitamin D levels. This can be followed up at regular intervals.

Studies[15] have found quantitatively that lower than optimum levels of concentration of active vitamin D corresponded to weak regulation of the immune response where - once a pathogen/antigen enters the body - the nature of the immune

---

[15] https://arxiv.org/abs/1304.7193

response would be less regulatory and hence, more aggressive or inflammatory. The immune system responding to this invasion, starts producing effector T-cells. These are cells which are involved in the body's defences. Generally, many more effector T cells than are needed are produced. It appears that the immune system goes into overdrive. Unfortunately, these effector T cells don't always distinguish between what is foreign material and what isn't. As such, effector T cells may start destroying their own body tissues. If this scenario occurs in the brain neuro-inflammation occurs which can eventually lead to neurodegeneration.

Optimum vitamin D levels reduce this hyperactivity which affects effector T cells. This hyperactivity also affects cells known as Antigen Presenting Cells (APC). One of these APC's - the microglial cell - is implicated in autoimmunity and neurodegeneration.

The microglia – which are 'mopping up' lymphocytes appear to be out of control in MND and have been described as the 'wind fanning the flames in the progression of MND. As the majority of people are vitamin D deficient for various reasons, a contributory factor for the progression of MND may well be a lack of available vitamin D.

Studies show that there is a greater likelihood of being diagnosed with MND for those taking statins than those who aren't on statins.[16] One possible reason for this is an

---

[16] *Amyotrophic Lateral Sclerosis Associated with Statin Use: A Disproportionality Analysis of the FDA's Adverse Event Reporting System.* It was published by the journal *Drug Safety* in April of 2018.

insufficient supply of cholesterol which is required for the maintenance of neural tissues. The knock on effect of this is simply that vitamin D can only be synthesised from the action of sunlight on the cholesterol which is found just below the skin's surface. Therefore, insufficient cholesterol will jeopardise the synthesis of vitamin D which helps regulate microglia so that they don't attack 'self' tissue. I will discuss this, and statins, in more detail later since statins impact on the synthesis of substances which are essential for neuro health as well as general health.

Those people who are particularly likely to be at risk of a vitamin D deficiency.

Older People – because:

Skin gets thinner as you get older. This makes it harder to make Vitamin D when it is exposed to sunlight.

- Older people tend to eat less and also tend to spend more time indoors – both these will reduce the amount of vitamin D someone has in their system.

People with Darker Skin because:

- The melanin in their skin helps protect them from the sun's ultra violet rays which reduces the body's ability to make this vitamin from the sun.

People with medical conditions that reduce fat absorption and those on low fat diets because:

- Vitamin D is fat soluble and needs a properly functioning gut to be able to absorb fat from the diet. As vitamin D is fat soluble it cannot be found in foods which don't contain fat. People who may be affected include those with Crohn's disease and liver disease.

Those who live further away from the equator or work indoors because:

- They are exposed to less sunlight.

Those on cholesterol lowering drugs such as statins because:

- Cholesterol is required to make vitamin D

Dietary sources of Vitamin D

- Cod Liver Oil: one tablespoon contains approximately 1,400 international units. In the shorter months - from October until March - I would recommend two tablespoons daily for anyone with a neurodegenerative disease or who belong to the susceptible groups already mentioned above.

- Cooked salmon: three ounces contains about 450 international units
- Beef liver: three ounces contains about 40 international units
- Egg yolk: one large, 40 international units[17]
- Irradiated mushrooms: three ounces, 35 international units.

---

[17] *Irradiated mushrooms have been left out in the sun and absorb ultra violet rays.

As you can appreciate, it is difficult, if not impossible to take in up to 4000 IU's of vitamin D, daily, through diet.

Vitamin E – An Essential Vitamin for Brain Health.

Vitamin E (tocopherol) is a fat soluble vitamin which is *essential* for optimum brain health. It has antioxidant properties which means that it can prevent or stop cell damage. Several neurodegenerative diseases, including MND are associated with oxidative stress. Antioxidants such as vitamin E reduce this load and, in doing so, slow down the progression of the disease. A 2011 clinical trial[18] showed that high-dose Vitamin E may help slow progression of ALS. The recommended dosage is 500mg twice daily.

---

[18] http://alsworldwide.org/care-and-support/article/supplements-and-vitamins

Sources of Vitamin E

- Seeds especially almonds

- Oils (especially wheat germ oils which are not found in white bread)

- Dark green leafy vegetables (taken with a little butter to aid absorption of this fat soluble vitamin).

Vitamin A

Vitamin A is a fat soluble vitamin and is found in many brain healthy fats such as butter, oily fish and egg yolk. It is found in large quantities in liver and there is a precursor of vitamin A – carotene – which is found in orange coloured vegetables such as carrots and, pumpkin.

Retinoic acid is the bioactive metabolite of Vitamin A. It modulates neurogenesis, neuronal survival and synaptic plasticity. [19] In other words, it helps keep neuronal cells healthy.

---

[19] Mol Nutr Food Res. 2010 Apr;54(4):489-95. doi: 10.1002/mnfr.200900246.
Significance of vitamin A to brain function, behavior and learning.

Olson CR[1], Mello CV.

The Necessity for Cholesterol in Maintaining Good Brain Health

Cholesterol has a bad press - like full fat milk, butter and egg yolks they've all been unfairly demonised. Anyone with a suggestion of a 'high' serum cholesterol level is generally offered statins in an effort to artificially lower their levels. Many others – and I know quite a few of these individuals – are given statins, when their cholesterol levels (and blood pressure levels) are within current acceptable levels[20], as a preventative measure. The body, at that point, appears to be healthy.
If statins are taken when there is no need for them, the effect will be to reduce cholesterol levels below that which is required for health.

Cholesterol has numerous functions in the body and is a **vital ingredient** for brain structure. By not supplying enough cholesterol, one of the potential outcomes is neurodegeneration and an inability to repair any injury to neural tissue.

Cholesterol is a waxy substance which our bodies make naturally and further, makes it in far greater quantity than we take in through our diet. The body MAKES WHAT IT NEEDS. If we take in more cholesterol through food than we require our body will adjust and make less. It does not blindly churn it out

---

[20] Cholesterol levels were based on what was common' for Americans. The concentration results are plotted on histograms and the type of distribution established. The reference ranges are derived from the central 95th percentile.

willy nilly, day after day, regardless of how much, or little, is required.

I have spoken to many people who have had a blood test to check their cholesterol levels and who have subsequently been informed that their cholesterol levels are too high. They have been advised to take statins. Some have refused to do so and unfortunately a fairly high percentage have been informed that if they refuse to take statins then they will need to find another GP. Others have been offered one further blood test to ascertain whether their cholesterol levels are still high. This suggests to me that clinicians are aware of the fluctuating nature of cholesterol. When the offer has been taken up, it has been found that the level of cholesterol has lowered itself naturally without any medical intervention or the need for statins... How or why has this happened?

Serum levels of many substances, including cholesterol will vary depending on what has been recently eaten. A high cholesterol meal which might include prawns, for example, will increase serum cholesterol levels temporarily. If a blood test is taken shortly after the prawns have been eaten, then serum levels may appear abnormally high. A healthy functioning liver, however, is very efficient at bringing levels down to what are optimum levels for the body at the time, so it is only a temporary and easily adjustable event. However, within this lies another tale.

Studies have also shown that stress contributes to a rise in cholesterol levels but quickly drops back once the stressful event is over. There is no great mystery about this – cholesterol is used in the formation of hormones including adrenaline. Adrenaline is needed to assist the body in coping with stress. Adrenaline is made in the adrenal medulla of the adrenal glands and also in some neurons. Cholesterol has to travel to these target organs from the liver where it is made. Its transport system in the circulatory system so at times of stress when more adrenalin is required, then there will be a corresponding increase in serum cholesterol. This is not an abnormal response. It is an adaptive response.

At any point in time the body's demands for cholesterol may rise. It may be that an extra fat laden meal is eaten in which case extra bile is required. To accommodate this short term event, serum cholesterol will rise as the body responds to the challenge of producing more bile. In fact, serum cholesterol levels may differ markedly throughout the day. The rhythmic rise and fall of serum cholesterol should not be a cause of concern.

Some of the vital processes which cholesterol is involved in are:

- Making bile which is required to process and digest fat.
- Making hormones such as oestrogen, adrenal hormones and testosterone.
- It is required for the production of insulation around nerve cells (the myelin sheath).
- Cholesterol is converted to Vitamin D by sunlight. Vitamin D is required for many processes in the body including the health of the brain and bones.
- It builds the structure of cell membranes

- Cholesterol is required to form memories. Information on the leaflets accompanying statins state that taking statins may cause memory loss.

My research, which I undertook some time ago, showed the dangers of lowering cholesterol by taking statins. This piece of research – a literature review - showed

- Higher levels of cholesterol are correlated with longevity.
- Low serum cholesterol is correlated with higher mortality.
- A 1mg fall of cholesterol in every dl of serum increased mortality by approximately 14% annually
- Those people with higher low density lipoprotein (supposedly the bad cholesterol) had better memories than those with low levels. In fact, research has established that there are higher rates of dementia in those individuals with low levels of cholesterol in comparison to those who have what would be considered high levels.
- In spite of popular belief, cholesterol has never been clinically proven to be the causative factor of any heart attack and further, more than three quarters of individuals who have a heart attack have normal levels of cholesterol.
- Low levels of cholesterol are a clinically proven risk factor for a number of different types of cancer as well as respiratory and gastro intestinal diseases.

- Cholesterol supports the immune system by improving signalling in a set of cells known as Tregs. This helps fight inflammation. Studies have shown that increased Tregs slows down the progression of motor neurone disease and other neurodegenerative disorders.
- Coffee intake has also been found to slow down the progression of MND. It is interesting to note that the intake of coffee is correlated with an increase in cholesterol levels – about 10%.
- Cholesterol helps absorb fat soluble vitamins ADEK
- It helps take up serotonin in the brain. Serotonin is a neurotransmitter which aids sleep
- Foods containing cholesterol are the main dietary sources of choline. This B vitamin is essential for the health of the liver, brain and nervous system.

It is clear that if cholesterol levels are artificially lowered through the use of medication that one or more of the areas which require cholesterol for optimum health are going to suffer.

Research continues to demonstrate that those with higher cholesterol levels have greater longevity, better memories and overall health, including more structurally healthy brains and nervous tissue. The cell body wall is made from cholesterol without which cells would collapse and die.

The Framingham Heart Study which was a huge piece of research found that statins did not benefit anyone over the age of 47 and found that those with higher levels of cholesterol lived longer.

What is perhaps most chilling is that researchers at the University of California and Advera Health Analytics inc worked together to analyse data from the FDA Adverse Event Reporting System (FAERS) to determine what is known as reporting odds ratios (RORS) involving statin drug users who have reported ALS symptoms.

An ROR of two means the risk is twice as higher. The determination of likelihood of statin user's increased risk for ALS by statin products as found to be thus

Statin Drug Name	–	ROR
Rosuvastatin		9.09 (809%)
Pravastatin		16.2 (1,502%)
Atorvastatin		17.0 (1,600%) *
Simvastatin		23.0 (2,200%) *
Lovastatin		107 (10,600%)

Table showing RORS for developing ALS type symptoms for specific statins.

Most statisticians consider an ROR above six as a likely cause of presenting symptoms associated with ALS.

Foods which are high in cholesterol

- Liver
- Kidneys
- Eggs
- Prawns

Before we go any further, it perhaps needs that HDL or LDL is NOT cholesterol. They are lipoproteins and are carriers for cholesterol. There isn't any 'good' or 'bad' cholesterol. Cholesterol is cholesterol regardless of whether it is carried on the LDL raft or the HDL raft.

The above four foods mainly known for their high cholesterol are actually fairly low in saturated fat. However, as we shall see later it is not saturated fat that is a culprit in clogging up arteries -whether cardiac or neural ones. Saturated fat has been found in studies, to upregulate the 'good' HDL and the 'good' LDL (yes there is a beneficial low density lipoprotein!) It is this LDL which carries the cholesterol which helps form memories and transports nutrients to cells. Without this LDL our cells would starve and with it the beginnings of neurodegeneration would occur as the cells die. Microglia, among other immune system cells would be directed to mop up dead and dying cells.

Blood tests for cholesterol do not take into account the positive impact that LDL-A has on the health of cells, as a whole, in addition to the positive benefits it has on memory.

There is a supposedly rogue LDL known as LDL-C, which is smaller and denser, than the good LDL but studies do not support the warnings that it is inherently atherosclerotic. In fact, studies show that this LDL too, is correlated with increased longevity.[21]

The Framingham heart study found that after the age of forty-seven, it made no difference whether a man's cholesterol was high or low in relation to a risk for heart disease.

William Castelli M.D. wrote this which appeared in the Archives of Internal medicine.

In Framingham Mass., the more saturated fat one ate, the more cholesterol one ate, the more calories one ate, the lower the person's serum cholesterol .... we found that people who ate the most cholesterol, ate the most saturated fat [and] ate the most calories, weighed the least and were the most physically active.

IN spite of numerous well designed, peer reviewed studies, statins continue to be doled out as a preventative medicine when, in fact, they are not preventing heart disease, they are setting up the seeds of a neurodegenerative disorder. The sharp rise in ALS which occurred in the 1990's, also coincided with the time when statins were heavily marketed.

---

[21] https://bmjopen.bmj.com/content/6/6/e010401

Plant based foods do not contain cholesterol and lower cholesterol levels when eaten. Since cholesterol's demonization, manufacturers have jumped onto the band wagon and produced a range of margarines and yogurt type drinks which promise to lower cholesterol levels thus preying on the ignorance of people about the importance of this substance. People are paying grossly inflated prices to damage their health!

Lowering cholesterol levels, through the use of statins, has not been proven to have prevented even one heart attack. High cholesterol levels are associated with increased longevity and impacts positively on the structure and function of the brain. Cholesterol, for example, has a critical role to play in the transmission of neurotransmitters. This means they pass messages on. Acetylcholine, for example, which requires cholesterol for its formation, is necessary for motor control, learning, memory, sleep and dreaming.

The soluble fibre found in oatmeal, many fruits and lentils, for example is applauded as being able to reduce levels of cholesterol. It does this because it is not absorbed in the intestine and so binds to cholesterol and removes it from the body. Once manufacturers realised that their products could reduce cholesterol, the prices of their goods went up. There appears to be an inverse correlation between the price of such goods and cholesterol related health benefits.

The more cholesterol is reduced the greater the likelihood of a neurodegenerative disorder, vitamin D deficiency and a whole host of problems stemming from its unavailability to perform its essential role in body and brain!

Cholesterol, heart disease and neurodegeneration

It is probably necessary at this point to introduce some facts about cholesterol and heart disease even though this book is for people with neurodegenerative disease, especially MND. This is because

- a great deal of research has been conducted on cholesterol and its perceived association with heart disease
- Those following an MND diet may be concerned about following a high fat and high cholesterol diet regardless of whether they have been placed on statins as a preventative measure for cardiovascular disease, or to bring down perceived dangerously high levels.

Some Facts

- 1953 Ancel Keys – biologist – proposed a radical theory that too much fat in the diet caused heart disease (Victorians who ate a very high fat diet had a very low incidence of heart disease but this passed him by).
- SEVEN COUNTIES STUDY - Ancel Keys looked at the connection between fat consumption and heart disease of 22 countries. He selected seven countries which fitted his hypothesis and discarded the rest.
- When concerned researchers looked at the evidence from **all of** the countries in the study they found that no association between high fat diets, cholesterol and heart disease existed.

- John Yudkin – British researcher – found that the ONLY dietary factor that had the strongest link to heart disease was **sugar.**
- British Physician – Mendrick - found that if he chose another seven different countries that the more saturated fat and cholesterol consumed the lower the risk of heart disease.
- THE FRAMINGHAM HEART STUDY - conducted over 16 years of over 5,000 people in Massachusetts. This study showed that those who had heart disease and those who didn't had similar ranges of cholesterol and lowering cholesterol levels for people who had heart disease only had any impact up to the age of forty-seven years. At the age of 48 years those with high cholesterol levels lived longer than those with low cholesterol levels. AND the more saturated fat, cholesterol and calories eaten, the lower the person's serum cholesterol was AND they were more physically active!
- Studies have shown that cholesterol neutralises toxins produced by bacteria. This may be why it is found at the site of arterial injuries. Of course some pathogens are able to cross the blood brain barrier, invade the brain, instigate neuro-inflammation and consequently neurodegeneration. Other pathogens which normally do not cross the blood brain barrier may do so if the brain is damaged in some way. This is what we are wanting to avoid in the first place. Cholesterol helps protect and repair the brain if such damage due to injury or infection occurs.

Good Fats, Bad Fats

Saturated fats are those fats which are solid at room temperature – butter, lard, dripping, meat and coconut oil are examples of saturated fat.

Saturated fats are another substance which have become demonised even though studies show that they raise HDL. Saturated fat also changes the pattern of LDL, increasing the subgroup of LDL which transports much needed substances for cell growth and repair. Studies have shown that saturated fat is associated with less coronary atherosclerosis than it if it is replaced by other food groups. When saturated fat is replaced with carbohydrate, for example, then the progression of atherosclerosis is greater. Further, when saturated fats are replaced with unsaturated fats, the progression of atherosclerosis also increases.

Saturated fat has many advantages over other fats for cooking. It is far more stable and so is less likely to be damaged when heated than, for example, oils such as olive oil or rape seed oil.

A further group of fats - The poly unsaturated fats - are the omega 6's, omega 3's, docosahexaenoic acid (DHA) and eicosapentoic acid (EPA).

The polyunsaturated acid found in omega six is called linoleic acid. It is derived from vegetable oils and it is a major player in fuelling inflammatory processes. Neurodegeneration and inflammation go hand in hand. Our diet is full of omega 6 without us realising it. These vegetable oils are added to just about every food on the market. It is hidden in biscuits and cakes, added to tinned soups etc., it is now used for cooking fish and chips in when once lard was used.

Lard could be considered a superfood. It is the second richest source of Vitamin D and is rich in cholesterol. It does not contain trans-fat – the real culprit behind heart disease –and contains 60% monounsaturated fat which is associated with a decreased risk of heart disease. Monounsaturated fats also decrease inflammation. This is one of our prime tasks in the fight against neurodegeneration.

Monounsaturated fats help promote a healthy blood flow to the brain. They help to produce and release acetylcholine which is essential for learning and memory; the loss of acetylcholine will result in memory problems often associated with Alzheimer's disease.

Most of the population are not aware of how much ubiquitous pro-inflammatory oil they are ingesting. When it comes to saturated fat and omega 6, it cannot be repeated enough that the latter creates inflammation. Studies show that it is the balance between omega 6 and omega three which impacts far more on health than saturated fat. We should be eating far more omega 3 in our diet than we currently are and the amount of omega 6's should be limited significantly, if they have to be used.

Omega 3 contains alpha linoleic acid which is found in walnuts and flaxseeds. It is anti-inflammatory and there should be about six times the amount of omega 3's ingested to the omega 6's. The reality is that it is the other way around. We are eating far too many vegetable oils containing the pro-inflammatory omega 6. In other words, we are providing the fuel for a state of chronic inflammation including neurodegeneration.

Earlier, I mentioned that the Victorians suffered very little heart disease in spite of their high saturated fat diet which was full of lard, dripping, eggs and butter. In fact, heart disease wasn't considered important enough to study at medical school in those times, since there was so little of it.

Eventually these important saturated fats were replaced with the 'healthier' substitutes of.

- Omega 6 vegetable oils
- margarine

I shall return to the subject of vegetable oils and margarine later.

> Eggs were demonised as being full of 'bad' cholesterol. People were frightened to eat one of the most nutritionally and complete foods to be found. The 'Go to work on an egg' was replaced by messages that eggs contained salmonella and should be avoided. The junior minister – Edwina Currie – eventually had to resign from her post after the British Egg Industry Council called her remarks 'factually incorrect and highly irresponsible' saying that the risk of

being infected with salmonella was less than 200 million to one.

Since saturated fats were replaced with 'healthier' substitutes, heart disease and neurodegenerative disease have increased markedly. Further, the introduction of cholesterol lowering drugs – which occurred more or less at the same time as these dietary changes - provide cogent explanations for the increase in chronic diseases.

Dr Weil M.D. in his book Healthy Aging observed that during the plenary presentations of the 11th Anti-Aging Conference and Exposition that it was mooted that chronic inflammation was a common root of neuro-degenerative disorders including Alzheimer disease, Parkinson's disease and Amyotrophic Sclerosis. It was emphasised that dietary modifications were a treatment strategy – a view point which I also hold. However, it is unlikely to be promoted as a treatment strategy. It does not hold any profit for the pharmaceutical companies.

The Macronutrient Choline

Choline is a recently discovered macronutrient which has some similarities with the Vitamin B complex. Both support brain function. It has numerous important roles in the body - functions which are carried out repeatedly on a daily basis. These include

- Optimum liver function
- Normal brain development and
- nerve function (nerve signalling) as it is a component of acetylcholine – a neurotransmitter - which helps nerves to communicate and muscles to
- move
- Healthy metabolism
- Supporting energy levels
- It is involved in methylation which is used to create DNA
- It is used in detoxification

Choline is a structural component of fat and is found in foods which contain natural fats. However, it is a water soluble macronutrient. Small amounts of choline are made in the liver but these small amounts are not nearly enough to make up what is considered to be the acceptable intake.

Choline and the neurotransmitter acetylcholine are both involved in a rechargeable chemical cycle. As an impulse reaches a motor end plate the nerve ending releases acetylcholine which instigates events in the muscle cell.

When the muscle contracts another substance called cholinesterase begins breaking down the accumulated acetylcholine and clearing it away. This allows for the next arriving nerve impulse to set the cycle in motion again.

There are approximately one thousand single impulses a second which could not take place without adequate amounts of choline. As choline is generally found in foods which contain natural fats it can be seen that our love affair with very low fat or no fat diets is not conducive to good brain function.

Dietary sources of choline and acceptable intake

As choline has only recently been discovered, a recommended dietary allowance has not been established. However, an agreed acceptable intake is approximately 450-550 mg daily.

Choline is found naturally in cauliflower, broccoli, Brussels sprouts, salmon, eggs, liver, beef and breast milk.

Table 1

Some food sources of choline

Food	Mg per Serving
Beef liver 3 ounces	360mg
One large egg	145mg
Braised beef 3 ounces	117mg
Chicken breast 3 ounces	77mg
Cod 3 ounces	71mg
One large baked potato	57mg
Soybeans half a cup	110mg
Kidney beans	45mg
One cup milk	43mg
Half a cup of dried, roasted peanuts	24mg

Other foods – mainly vegetables – contain smaller amounts of this macronutrient. As you can appreciate, a 'typical' diet is unlikely to contain the Acceptable Daily Intake especially if eggs have been removed in an effort – however mistakenly - to maintain a heart healthy diet. Further, liver is not a popular food now, yet it contains a wealth of nutrients essential for brain health including, more or less, all the choline required daily, in one small portion.

It may be worth jotting down what you eat over one day to ascertain whether the diet provides anywhere near the Acceptable Intake of 450-550mg of choline daily. Fortunately, where tastes, or lack of appetite, mean that the Acceptable Intake is unlikely to be consistently reached, this macronutrient can be obtained at all good health food stores.

Vitamin B Complex

This complex consists of 8 vitamins: B1, B2, B3, B5, B6, B7, B9 and B12. They are water soluble vitamins. Some of these will be looked at individually below.

The effect of the B vitamins on neurological health is wide ranging. Some of this complex's functions impact on

- The maintenance of the myelin sheath which is a fatty sheath which surrounds nerve cells. Without this fatty coating, nerve signalling is impaired and affects motor function, cognition and mood.
- The Methylation Cycle
- The production and function of neurotransmitters

Vitamin B1 (Thiamine) – Thiamine was first discovered in 1926. It works synergistically with B2 and B6. It is easily destroyed by cooking, caffeine, food processing, alcohol and some drugs. Some studies have shown that lack of thiamine results in

- Poor or absent nerve impulses as it plays an essential role in nerve impulses
- Thiamine ensures that the brain and nerves have enough glucose for their requirements
- Studies have shown that thiamine deficiency has been shown to reduce the diameter of myelinic fibres as well as *increase cell death in the brain.*

Good Sources of Thiamine

- Wholemeal grain
- Liver
- Eggs
- Pork
- Fish
- Nuts
- Green vegetables

Vitamin B3 (Niacin) – Niacin is necessary to maintain a healthy circulation to the brain. This helps maintain concentration and focus. It is also a potent antioxidant and scavenges the free radicals which can set off neuro-inflammation. In the preface of this book I mentioned that microglia are cells in the brain which mop up inflammation and diseased cells. An excess of microglia appears to be the 'wind fanning the flames' in the progression of MND. An adequate intake of niacin can therefore reduce the potential for inflammation in the first place and avoid rapid progression of MND and other forms of neurodegeneration.

Interestingly, *studies have also shown that quercetin and resveratrol reduced neuronal cell death instigated by microglial activation* suggesting that they are potent anti-inflammatory compounds. We shall look at quercetin in more detail, later.

Resveratrol is found in red wine and grapes. The latter is the preferred form for taking in resveratrol since alcohol is toxic to the brain.

.

How niacin deficiency has the potential to lead to brain cell death.

Niacin is a forerunner to two coenzymes. Coenzymes are just non protein substances which are essential for enzymes to function. These coenzymes are abbreviated to NAD and NADP.

NAD is needed to break down large substances into smaller ones. In this case it breaks down fats, carbohydrates and proteins into much smaller units.

NAD is also used to repair DNA and is involved in cell signalling.

NAD can convert to NADH and by a number of processes transfers food from diet into energy. If it is not required, it is stored as ATP.

ATP fuels the mitochondria which are the powerhouses in each cell. The mitochondria produce the energy with which we need to survive. If there isn't enough NADH then ATP will become depleted. Neuronal cell death is a potential outcome of this.

Vitamin B6 (Pyroxidone)

Pyroxidone helps make neurotransmitters and the protein, haemoglobin, which helps transport oxygen around the blood.

 B6 is probably better known for maintaining normal levels of homocysteine which is an amino acid in the blood. High levels of homocysteine are associated with cardiovascular disease. In spite of this I have never known patients to be informed that it is homocysteine which is a contributory for heart disease rather than cholesterol. This is not surprising given that a month's supply of vitamin B complex can be bought for as little as £2-£3 pounds off the supermarket shelf and cannot make profits for pharmaceutical companies in the way that statins can and do.

Vitamin B9 (Folic Acid) – studies undertaken at the University of Wisconsin, Madison on rats, suggests that folic acid may help promote healing in injured brains and spinal cord.

Vitamin B12 (Cobalamin) – this vitamin is essential for the development and function of brain and nerve cells. It helps promote the synthesis of lecithin which is a major component of the myelin sheath lipids.

There are only animal sources of Vitamin B12 and even then, this vitamin can only be separated from its food source in an acidic environment. Stomach acidity tends to reduce in older age and further many elderly people take antacids which both impact on how well vitamin B12 can be absorbed. Further problems arise when there is loss of appetite often associated with illness and old age.

Studies have shown ***marked increases in T regulatory cells*** after vitamin B12 supplementation. It is this increase in T regulatory cells which has been shown to slow down the rate of progression of MND.

Vitamin B complex and the perils of smoking.

The vitamin B complex is easily destroyed by smoking which especially impacts vitamin B12. Strangely enough studies have found that large doses of vitamin C also destroy vitamin B12. The vitamin B complex is better taken first thing in the morning when vitamin C rich meals are less likely to be taken. Further, it produces energy – something which you do not need a great deal of when you are trying to sleep.

Sources of Vitamin B complex in food

As stated vitamin B12 is only found in animal sources – meat, fish, dairy and eggs. Vegetarians and vegans are therefore, especially at risk of vitamin B12 deficiency.

Other forms of this B complex are generally found in meat, eggs, dairy and wholemeal foods such as bread, oats, and wheat germ. It is often added to breakfast cereals.

It is possible to be deficient in this complex given that it is so easily destroyed through a number of avenues.

Anyone with a neurodegenerative disorder should automatically have their B12 levels tested.

Given the importance of vitamin B complex in brain health, I would always recommend taking it in tablet form in addition to obtaining it from food although this complex is often added to cereals. It can be destroyed by cooking and is water soluble and is likely to leach out of foods when cooking. Needs for many nutrients rise when an individual is unwell but often appetite fails. It can be found in supermarkets and is inexpensive.

Vitamin C (ascorbic acid)

Most people are familiar with vitamin C. It has antioxidant properties and helps to reduce inflammation.

Vitamin C is found in fresh fruit and vegetables but it is water soluble and it is also easily destroyed by sunlight and when food is cooked. A large orange will provide enough vitamin C for an individual's daily needs but this rises during periods of illness, stress and injury.

Large quantities of vitamin C can cause diarrhoea and in some cases vitamin C can act as a pro-inflammatory. With this in mind, supplementation is generally not necessary.

The Connection between MND, Exercise and Glutamic Acid

Research has already found an association between exercise and the increased likelihood of developing MND. What has not been established is how the two are linked together.

Firstly, I will be using similar terms throughout this chapter such as glutamic acid, glutamate and glutamine. These terms can be used interchangeably. They are all forms of one amino acid which is absolutely essential for the health of the brain and muscle. The differences only lie in where these can be found in the body and their own specific functions. Thus

- Glutamic acid is generally found in the brain
- Glutamate is the form which is a neurotransmitter – essential for passing messages along nerves to their target organ
- Glutamine is found in the brain and the body. It is especially concentrated/stored in the muscles.

Normally there is enough glutamic acid in the diet to meet an individual's needs. However, in times of stress such as exercise or the stress associated with medical conditions or poor nutritional status, to name but a few, an individual's requirements for glutamic acid rises. Thus, glutamic acid is called a conditional amino acid which means that normally an individual can make what they need but in times of stress, extra will be required. Athletes know the importance of glutamic acid for they supplement with this amino acid during workouts. During intense exercise the body's levels of glutamic acid can decrease by as much as 60%.

Glutamic acid is essential for the health of the skin and when levels are low then it is simply withdrawn from the muscle store leaving them weak, stringy and unable to perform their function properly.

Every part of the body, including the brain, breaks down worn out proteins and builds up new replacement ones, provided the right building blocks are available.

When protein degradation occurs – a catabolic state – ammonia is released. Ammonia is highly toxic to the brain and instigates inflammatory processes. This may result in sick cells and ultimately cell death. However, in the presence of a sufficient supply of glutamic acid, ammonia is neutralised by combining with it and forming the harmless glutamine.

Post exercise, there may not be a sufficient supply of glutamic acid available. This allows ammonia to begin to wreak havoc on delicate neurons through the inflammatory process.

Chronic inflammation may continue for some time before initial symptoms of a neurodegenerative disorder (NDD) manifests itself. The individual may continue following a 'healthy' lifestyle in the form of long walks, a low fat/no fat diet and take statins as a preventative measure. Food intake consists of salads and low fat veggies with little protein – hardly a recipe to increase glutamic acid levels which are vital for the health of so many structures and processes in the body. In this scenario – which is a part of so many people's lives nowadays – we have everything set up to instigate neurodegeneration and all in the name of a 'healthy' lifestyle.

The only prescribed medication – Riluzole – which is purported to slow down the rate of progression of MND by reducing the amount of glutamic acid available in the brain, appears to work in the opposite way to that which appears to promote brain health.

The reasoning behind the conception of Riluzole was that it reduced the production of a neuro excitatory neurotransmitter – glutamate – which is stated could be toxic in large amounts to brain cells. There appeared to be little consideration of the fact that glutamic acid is a precursor for gamma amino butyric acid (GABA) which is an inhibitory neurotransmitter. Therefore, by artificially reducing glutamic acid

- Neutralisation of ammonia – which is a highly toxic substance to the brain – may not occur.
- Cognitive brain dysfunctions may occur
- GABA production may not be adequate and as a result its qualities of tranquillity, improved concentration and improved sleep may be denied the patient.
- It is able to pass through the blood brain barrier and, as such, is one of the brain's primary 'foods,' when available.
- It has been used as a treatment for schizophrenia, Parkinson's disease, muscular dystrophy and alcoholism, among others.

Given the above, it is madness to mess with the production of a conditional amino acid. (By conditional, we mean that that the body is able to produce what it needs apart from at times of stress or injury when supplementation may be necessary). However, what is happening is, that once MND had been diagnosed - which indicates a higher need for glutamic acid given, for example, that the inflammatory processes will result in cell degradation and increased release of ammonia - Riluzole which reduces the production of glutamic acid is offered.

Recent research shows the lack of efficacy of Riluzole. Further, the MNDA state in their literature that

[3] *The anti-glutamate effect may be a reason why it provides some benefit for people with MND, <u>but this is not yet proven.</u>*

The use of Riluzole is said to increase life expectancy by 2-4 months although **there is currently no evidence to support this statement.** Further, Glutamate increases Tregs and may have a protective role in inflammatory and neurodegenerative disorders. This is a desired outcome.

It perhaps needs repeating that the upregulation of Tregs is associated with a slower progression of MND yet Riluzole reduces the amount of glutamate which is synthesised. In addition, glutamate has been found to have potent effects on cancer and autoimmune pathological T cells. Glutamate receptors have been found on immune system cells – T cells, B cells, macrophages and dendritic cells which suggests that it has a role in both the innate and adaptive immune system and restrains neuro-inflammation).

Glutamate is also essential for bone health and in the form of glutamic acid helps to maintain the moisture balance of the skin. Glutamate does not cross the blood brain barrier- unless it has been compromised through injury – and must be made inside the neurons from glutamine which is the by- product of ammonia and glutamic acid.

In rat models, increasing leucine – an amino acid – assists glutamate entry into the brain. This has been shown to restore brain function after injury. Further, studies have shown that glutamate derived from food activates the vagus nerve encouraging gut motility by increasing the serotonin levels in the gut. It also helps to maintain body heat.

When glutamic acid **is the only way the brain employs to detoxify the brain then it is simply madness to reduce levels through the use of medication.** Not only does glutamic acid remove waste ammonia, it also boosts the synthesis of glutathione, a powerful antioxidant, in addition to contributing to the health of the digestive system, immune system as well as being involved in energy production.

Aggression is also common in those with low levels of glutamic acid and GABA (gamma- amino-butyric acid).

Although there is no evidence to support the idea that Riluzole slows down the progression of MND, it continues to be prescribed. However, another substance – coffee - which **has** been proven to slow down the rate of progression of MND, has not even been included in the dietary recommendations for those with MND. I find this bewildering.

What is happening here? Drugs are constantly brought to market purporting to help with certain conditions. Often these conditions are terminal or impact greatly on people's lives such that individuals will grasp at anything offered, even if there is no evidence that it works. Maybe the extra two months of life that Riluzole is said to offer (not evidenced), is simply a placebo effect. However, its prescribing does make profits for pharmaceutical companies.

Meanwhile, coffee – whether with caffeine or not, has been researched and proven to slow down the rate of progression of MND. This is not surprising considering it contains powerful brain antioxidants. Is this marvellous drug and its effects given space in literature? No!

The cynics among us – and I am one of them – might just believe that, as there isn't any profit in marketing coffee as a treatment for MND, so its potential benefits aren't laid before those who have been diagnosed with this disease.

Here we have some evidence that antioxidants support brain health and slow down progression of degenerative diseases. Yet we aren't building on this. We have swept this aside and produced a drug with unproven effects, which may ultimately have a detrimental effect on the brain.

Of course, it would be ideal if everyone knew the importance of glutamic acid during periods of physical stress etc. but unfortunately this knowledge appears to be the preserve of the professional athletes. This appears to be true even though the level of intensity between professional athletes and those who are not, may differ little in the impact such activity has on glutamic acid levels. How often have I seen groups of young people out on walking holidays take out a salad sandwich and a Kendal mint cake for their lunch after a morning of hard walking – a meal which lacks any glutamic acid worth considering? As such, the seeds of loss of muscle mass and brain deterioration are in the making.

Any, or a combination, of the factors below has a potential to increase the risk of NDD

- Walking regularly including walking holidays
- Intense physical work such as work outs in the gym, heavy gardening
- Medical conditions, injury, accidents
- Stress of any form
- Poor nutritional status

Can the brain repair itself?

Myelin sheath is capable of rebuilding itself – this is demonstrated particularly with those who have multiple sclerosis (MS) – another neurodegenerative disorder – which involves both sensory and motor neurons. The catabolism of myelin sheath results in symptoms of a relapse, but repair will result in subsequent remission. As time goes by the relapsing-remitting type of MS often progress to secondary progressive MS. Nevertheless, during those two positions, repair does take place.

In order for the brain and its associated structures to give themselves the best possible chance of repairing themselves, the inflammatory processes need to be calmed and preferably eliminated. Research has demonstrated that the upregulation of thymus derived cells (Tregs) is associated with a reduction in inflammation and a slowing of the rate of the progression of MND. Further, the right building blocks in the form of amino acids, vitamins, minerals and fats have to be made available for use in this repair process... This means paying closer attention to diet as outlined in this book. There is no point in keeping to a no fat diet when the brain, and its structures, are composed mainly of fats. It would be impossible to rebuild/repair any areas which have been damaged by whatever means especially as vitamins ADEK are fat soluble and it is these which are essential for brain health.

Research has shown that treatment with sodium butyrate – found in butter, legumes and parmesan cheese, predominantly – supported the development of new nerve cells in the damaged areas of a stroke model (in mice). Therefore, the inclusion of these foods is highly recommended for those with a NDD including MND. The argument for replacing margarine and returning to good old butter will be looked at in more detail later.

Vitamin K - there is some limited research for this fat soluble vitamin supporting neuro health – again found in abundance in the dark green leafy vegetables – kale, chard etc.

Areas of the brain containing myelin have more K2 MK4. It is known as a key anti- aging vitamin.

How long does neuro repair take?

Different cells have different rates of turnover. Skin cells, for example, have a fairly rapid rate of turnover. A cut will have sealed itself with a scab and lost that scab by two weeks, leaving only a pink tell-tale mark to advertise that an injury ever occurred. Stomach cells take about 28 days to be replaced once shed. Neurons, however, can take up to a year to repair so any repair may not manifest itself immediately. This does not mean that regression to a previously unsuitable diet should occur. Patience is the key when it comes to a neurodegenerative disorder.

There are other factors which need to be taken into consideration in neuro repair. The earlier in the course of a disease that nutritional status can be upgraded, clearly has an impact on the amount of damage which we are trying, in part, to reverse. The time scale is also relevant when considering the breakdown of muscle tissue caused by insufficient glutamic acid, statins or steroids - among others - which are known to break down muscle tissue in a process called rhabdomyolysis.

Is rhabdomyolysis reversible? Research papers on this subject differ vastly. Some studies – and unfortunately those in the majority – have not found reversibility. However, a limited number of studies have found some. This is heartening but it begs the question whether the deemed irreversibility stemmed from not providing the right nutritional environment which would enhance the production of new muscle growth. Clearly, if poor nutritional status caused the breakdown of muscle fibres in the first place this needs to be corrected. If medication which may contribute rhabdomyolysis is currently prescribed, then an alternative should be sought which does not have this side effect.

There is a separate chapter in this book which looks at the negative impact which some medications have the potential to cause, on MND.

The case for using butter instead of margarine

Interest in how our gut functions and the good bacteria it supports, has developed in recent years. Further, there has been an emphasis on how diet impacts on the health of our brain. Most of this research is concerned with how fibre is tied up with the health of our colons but more recently this has included how butyrate – a short chain fatty acid (SCFA) which is produced by the fermentation of bacteria on fibre – has impacted positively on brain health.

Butyrate has a number of different actions and, as such, its chameleon like qualities are able to respond to a number of imbalances often found in neurological disorders. Further, studies[22] have found that the metabolism of a high fibre diet in the gut can alter gene expression in the brain which is able to prevent neurodegeneration, stop any further neurodegeneration occurring and, ultimately promote regeneration.

What has this got to do with using butter instead of margarine? Well, butyrate is a product of butyric acid. Butyric acid is found in abundance in butter - this is where butter gets its name from.

---

[22] https://www.gutmicrobiotaforhealth.com/en/can-high-fibre-diet-prevent-andor-treat-neurological-disorders/

It is highly recommended that if a butter substitute is normally used such as margarine, that this is replaced with butter.

Studies have shown that treatment with sodium butyrate, in mouse models, has supported the development of new nerve cells in areas damaged by stroke. Diets which are highly processed and rich in processed sugar result in low butyrate production as well as neuro inflammation. Highly processed diets result in the activation of microglia and astrocytes in the brain. This will promote neuronal loss and consequently disease progression.

And the perils of margarine and vegetable oils

Margarine was originally invented by a Frenchman in 1869. It was originally called oleomargarine. The 'oleo' from 'oleum' meaning 'beef' and the margarine meaning 'lustre.'

Margarine did not really become popular until the 1950's. In 1930. The average person ate over 18lb of butter and approximately 2lb of margarine.

Margarine was a cheap alternative to butter but there aren't any safe levels of trans fats. Trans fats are incorporated during the solidification of vegetable oil – most are which are made from omega -6 oils which are also highly inflammatory.

Margarine is formed from refined vegetable oils (linseed, rapeseed, palm, sunflower etc.) and water to which emulsifiers, salt, preservatives, buttermilk, vitamins and flavourings are added.

Margarine became part of people's diets more at the end of rationing when an even greater choice of brands became available. This was helped along by commercial TV advertising which came into being in 1955.

In the 1980's, perfectly healthful saturated fats were replaced by partially hydrogenated oils. The dangers of trans fats – if they were known – were ignored until much later. Most brands have stopped the use of hydrogenated oils and become trans-fat free. This took a while; Denmark was the first country to ban Tran's fats in 2003.

The oils which are very high in the inflammatory omega 6 are

- Sunflower
- Canola
- Rapeseed
- Corn
- Soybean
- Cottonseed

This is not an exhaustive list.

In 1900 there was much less cancer and heart disease than we have now. This has risen and coincides with the increase in the use of vegetable oil.

The normal fat content of the body is 97% saturated fat with the other 3% comprising 1.5% omega 6 oils and 1.5% omega three oils.

The saturated fats we used to eat in our diets has been replaced with 70१b of pro-inflammatory vegetable oil annually. It increased in 1950 when a governmental campaign was launched to encourage people to eat vegetable oils to avoid artery clogging saturated fats – this in spite of the lack of evidence that saturated fat clogged arteries.

We have only to look at the French way of eating – a diet which is rich in saturated fats such hard cheese and butter – and the well- known 'French paradox' to understand that saturated fat is not responsible for heart disease.

If this isn't evidence enough then the study from Western Ohio University may sway you. This study involved observing the impact of ten different dietary fats ranging from the most saturated to the least saturated. The diets rich in saturated fats produced the least number of cancers and the omega 6's the most. One of the reasons is that saturated fats do not break down to form free radicals. Vegetable oils, however, oxidise very easily and so they deplete the antioxidants in the body, very rapidly.

Oils which can be used freely

- Coconut – a source of medium chain fatty acids
- Butter
- Organic cream
- Palm oil - it is heat stable
- Olive oil – monounsaturated fatty acids
- Avocado oil
- Fish oil

Alpha Lipoic Acid

Alpha-lipoic acid is a powerful brain antioxidant and, as such, essential for brain health. It is a substance which is both fat and water soluble. It is found mainly in red meat – especially organ meats. There are only very small amounts to be found in vegetables. Therefore, those individuals who follow a vegetarian or vegan diet and who have been diagnosed with a neurodegenerative disorder need to consider supplementing their diet with this antioxidant. It is easily obtainable through health store outlets. Supplementing with alpha-lipoic acid may be a good protective strategy against neurodegeneration for anyone whose diet is more or less vegetable based.

Quercetin

Studies have shown that when microglia are activated then neuronal cell death has occurred. Studies have shown that quercetin has the ability to reduce neuronal cell death instigated by microglial activation. It is thought this is due to its powerful antioxidant properties.

Quercetin is mainly found in onions. Onions are a versatile vegetable and can be added to just about every savoury cooked dish as well tossed into salads or included in sandwiches. The type of onion does not matter.

A simple cheese on toast provides lots of nerve fibre building from the butyric acid in cheese and the fibre in wholemeal bread. The quercetin in the onions helps prevent neuronal loss. It is a good combination.

Avoiding weight loss with MND

The current thinking for those with MND is that weight must be maintained. Once lost, it is difficult to gain back. Most of the weight lost will most likely be due to the loss of muscle mass which requires protein for repair. However, recommendations for keeping weight stable is the addition of chocolate bars – or similar - which not only provide the highly processed diet that we are trying to avoid but also do little in terms of providing protein and retaining muscle mass. Highly processed foods are to be avoided as they support the inflammatory process.

When additional calories are required to maintain weight, then protein, complex carbohydrates and certain fats - which reduce neuro-inflammation – are the key players. Complex carbohydrates generally have the benefits of containing vitamin B complex which, as we've already discovered, is essential for brain health.

 Further, the brain is composed of approximately 60% fat so by increasing calorie intake through anti-inflammatory fats, we are not only helping to maintain weight but also contributing to the healthy structure of the cells found in the brain. The 'wrong' fats cannot be substituted in the diet with the hope that they will support brain structure and function. An analogy is that a house normally built with bricks cannot be adequate or fulfil its function if built using a substitute such as straw.

Whey protein is an excellent source of all the essential amino acids and can be added to water or milk and diluted to a consistency which makes it easier to swallow.

Whey protein can be found in most health food shops and comes in a number of flavours. The free form of whey protein needs no digesting at all. It is absorbed immediately and easily and can be added to cereals or soups, cake mixtures or sprinkled over food, if desired. There are non-flavoured varieties which adds to its versatility.

Salicylates

Salicylates are chemicals found in plants which have pain-relieving, anti-pyretic and anti-inflammatory properties. They are naturally occurring in many fruit and vegetables and help to protect plants from being attacked by fungus. Salicylates are also found in aspirin.

Studies have shown that aspirin might reduce the risk of ALS, and the benefit might be more prominent for older people.[23] The reason is thought to be because older people are more likely to take larger doses daily. Another study indicates that treatment with NSAID's, like aspirin, can restore brain cell production as well as lower levels of beta-amyloid by reducing inflammation. The latter is good news for those with Alzheimer's disease and other diseases which are fuelled by inflammation. While the number of neurons may increase, it does not necessarily mean that function is restored. The restoration of function has to be learned and is an entirely different process.

Other studies have shown similar findings in that salicylic acid-based treatments may help prevent excessive neuronal loss in neurodegenerative diseases. As such salicylates may have some

---

[23] Nov. 14 issue of *Science*, Dr. Steven Paul and researchers from the drug maker Eli Lilly and Co.

therapeutic value in treating or preventing many neurological diseases.

Aspirin has been found to be very effective at reducing free radicals by mopping them up in a very efficient manner. As free radicals injure and damage tissues then clearly reducing them is beneficial.

There are a number of downsides to taking aspirin and salicylates. Some of the side effects of aspirin are the potential for indigestion, gastritis and ulcers. Salicylates may cause allergy type symptoms, in susceptible people. These include

- Asthma like symptoms – wheezing and trouble breathing
- Headaches
- Nasal congestion
- Changes in skin colour
- Itching, skin rash and hives
- Swelling of the hands, feet and face
- Stomach pain

However, if aspirin and salicylates are not a problem then they can be included as a treatment to reduce the inflammation found in neurodegeneration.

Foods containing high amounts of salicylate are

Fruit

Blackberry, blackcurrant, apricots, blueberry, dates, grapes, orange, pineapple, plum, strawberry, prunes, raspberry and sultana

Vegetables

Chilli peppers, courgette, green olives, peppers, radish and water chestnut

Seeds and nuts

Almonds, peanuts with skins on

Honey

Herbs, spices and condiments

Coconut oil, olive oil, basil, bay leaf, caraway, chilli powder, nutmeg, vanilla essence

Buffered Soluble Aspirin similar to Alka Seltzer can be home made

2 uncoated aspirin

8 oz soda or sparkling water

1/2tsp baking soda

Juice from a wedge of lemon

This is not appropriate for a sodium restricted diet.

Nicotine

Several areas of the brain which are affected by Alzheimer's disease, mainly contain nicotine receptors for acetylcholine. However, the number of these receptors are greatly reduced. Acetylcholine is required for memory formation and so has a vital part to play in learning. It has been found that nicotine patches can aid memory.

Nicotine acts on the cholinergic system. The cholinergic system uses acetylcholine almost exclusively to send its messages. It is an agonist – a chemical that binds to a receptor and activates it to produce a biological response. An agonist causes an action to happen.

Nicotinic receptors are to be found throughout the nervous system and are involved in many physiological responses such as pain processing, feeding behaviour and cognitive functions. Dysfunctions of neuronal nicotinic receptors are implicated in many neurodegenerative disorders including MND, Alzheimer's disease and Parkinson's disease. There are also associations with autism spectrum conditions and schizophrenia.

High Fat Diets Increase Lifespan of individuals with ALS and other neurodegenerative disorders

A number of studies have identified that high carbohydrate and low fat intakes are associated with a higher ALS risk (Okamoto et al., 2007). Another epidemiologic study looked at the size and proportions of the body of the general population with a follow up over ten years. The conclusion was that a high fat content reduces the risk of developing ALS (Gallo et al., 2013). These clinical data are consistent with the reduced overall survival of SOD1 mice under caloric restriction. (Hamadeh et al 2005).

An event shed some light on the above. A group of scientists remained in an isolated environment and were subject to two years of caloric restriction (Watford et al, 2002). Out of eight members of the group, one died from ALS and another developed progressive gait impairment and motor neuron degeneration.

In contrast, increased energy intake is beneficial for SOD1 mice. Sod1 mice fed a diet enriched in lipids restored normal body mass and adiposity. It also delayed disease onset and motor neuron degeneration. Life expectancy was extended by 20% (Dupois et al, 2004). The benefits of a high fat diet or ketogenic diet need to be made known.

Another study found that dyslipidemia[24] defined by high LDL/HDL ratio was a characteristic of the ALS group (Dupois et al., 2008) and this dyslipidemia positively correlated with longer survival time increased by 13 months in the group of ALS patients with higher LDL/HDL ratio. This may well account for why there is a significantly increased risk for rapid progression of ALS in those who take statins.

Dorst et al 2011 found that either hyperlipidemia[25] or high body mass is a strong prognostic factor for survival. High serum triglyceride levels increased median life expectancy by 14

---

[24] Dyslipidemia in this case is an unexpected high LDL/HDL ratio which is generally frowned on but research shows actually has neuroprotective effects.
[25] Hyperlipidemia is the elevation of lipids in the blood above what would be expected

months and a lower LDL/HDL ratio has been linked to respiratory impairments (Chio et al 2009).

The **Ketogenic diet** has been in clinical use for nearly a century. It was used originally for the symptomatic treatment of epilepsy. Further, there is evidence that this diet may provide symptomatic and disease modifying activity in a broad range of neurodegenerative disease such as MND, Alzheimer's disease and Parkinson's disease. Studies in animal models show that ketone bodies, especially beta-hydroxybutyrate, confer neuroprotection against diverse types of cellular injury. The ketogenic diet appears to have a wide range of beneficial effects in a broad range of brain disorders characterised by the death of neurons.

The mechanisms of how this occurs are not yet fully understood. However, it is believed that the increased neuronal energy reserves assist neuronal ability to resist metabolic challenges. However, the possibility of increased antioxidant and anti-inflammatory effects cannot be ruled out.

The problem with medication

Many medications do not support the upregulation of T cells which is the desired outcome we are looking for if the rate of progression of MND is to be slowed. Some medications promote muscle breakdown and demyelination. Here are some of the culprit medications.

Bendroflumethiazide

This frequently prescribed diuretic appears fairly innocuous as most medications appear to be when they are commonly prescribed to the masses. However, studies show that

Bendroflumethiazide + exercise could = hyponatraemia and osmotic demyelination syndrome. Put more simply, this diuretic and exercise could cause the myelin sheath around nerve cells to break down. As the myelin sheath is essential for transmitting electrical impulses (messages) down the nerve, then anything which prevents it from doing its job will have profound effects on the individual's physical and ultimately, mental health.

Diuretics also have the potential to lower potassium levels and the consequences of this can be leukopenia – a condition which is the opposite of the upregulation of T cells. Diuretics, therefore, can indirectly progress the rate at which MND advances, through its action on potassium levels.

Hypokalaemia (low potassium, which is frequently caused by diuretics) also impacts negatively on muscle tissue and can cause rhabdomyolysis – breakdown of muscle tissue.

Statins and the mevalonate pathway

Most people will not have ever heard of the mevalonate pathway but without this pathway, and its synthesis of isoprenoids, cell rejuvenation could not occur. That is, cells die and cannot be replaced.

Cells are recycled at different rates. For example

- Gut cells are replaced every 10 hours to 5 days
- Skin cells turnover every two weeks
- Liver cells every 300-500 days
- Bone cells every decade

It can be seen that different parts of the body will suffer at different rates if the ability of the mevalonate pathway to rejuvenate cells, is blocked.

Some of the isoprenoids which are essential for cell energy and replication are

- Co enzyme Q10 – which provides cellular energy
- Heme A – vital for cell energy and drug metabolism

- Isoprentyl adenine – vital for DNA replication

The life of every cell in the human body is severely impaired by statins but which cells will be affected first depends on their turnover rate.

Diagram of the Mevalonate pathway

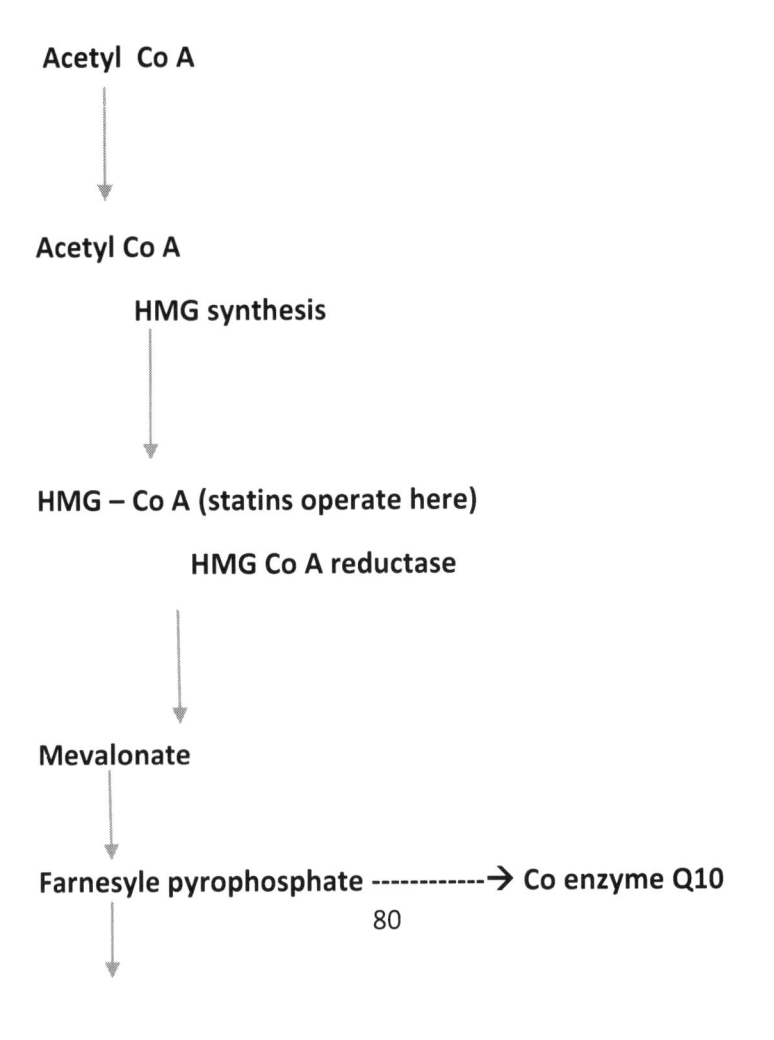

Acetyl Co A
↓

Acetyl Co A
    HMG synthesis
    ↓

HMG – Co A (statins operate here)
    HMG Co A reductase
    ↓

Mevalonate
↓

Farnesyle pyrophosphate ------------→ **Co enzyme Q10**
↓

Cholesterol

Statins are not just HMG – Co A reductase inhibitors – they are also reductase stimulators. That is, they will stimulate reductase production in an attempt to open the mevalonate pathway when cells, affected by statins, are dying.

The body only has two responses when cholesterol levels are too low to provide the body's needs. It can

- make more cholesterol but this option isn't open when statins are used
- take cholesterol from the blood stream. In this case the LDL receptor (LDL is not cholesterol just a carrier) works overtime grabbing LDL from the bloodstream to compensate for the fact that the cell cannot make as much. This means there is much less cholesterol in the bloodstream ready to respond to the cell's nutritional needs. As so many bodily functions depend on cholesterol, then cell death will occur.

Marvin Siperstein, in 1973 demonstrated that DNA replication was dependent on isoprenoids from mevalonate. However, statins block the synthesis of isoprenoids from mevalonate and without the ability to replicate, cells die.

In 1980 Brown and Goldstein co-authored a paper in The Journal of Biological Chemistry. In it they argued that Co A reductase was inhibited by a specific statin known as Compactin. Compactin blocks mevalonate and cultured cells died.

Cholesterol, by itself, is insufficient to prevent cell death although it is necessary for the health of a cell. However, even when mevalonate metabolites were added, they could not undo the damage from this statin.

Statins revisited – detrimental to brain health

Statins have already been discussed in some detail. However, studies have shown that they may negatively impact on NDD's such as ALS, dementia and Parkinson's disease.

An article by Scientific American has argued that some patients taking statins develop ALS or ALS-like conditions with progressive muscle wasting. In some – but not all – cases the condition may resolve once the medication has been stopped.

Many of the statin users who I have spoken to say that they have been to their GP's regarding muscle stiffness and pain. They are reassured – without further exploration of why this should be so – that it 'will not be the statins.' How can the medics be so sure?

Research has also shown the connection between statins and a greater incidence of developing type 2 diabetes. Type 2 diabetes will also impact negatively on the health of the brain as it is a systemic disease. It also impacts on muscle mass.

Statins and Co-enzyme Q10

Statins begin to exert their effects almost immediately. The symptoms brought about by statin use are generally slow and often put down to overwork, stress and age related joint pain. Some of these symptoms will be due to a statin's effect on levels of a co-enzyme known as Co-enzyme 10.

Co-enzyme Q10 is essential for neuromuscular function and respiration of cells. It has a role in energy transfer in skeletal muscle i.e. the muscle enabled by motor neurons. It also aids the development of all cells including neurons. Co-enzyme Q10 becomes depleted with age, illness and statin use and supplements may be necessary. Co-enzyme Q10 is found mainly in organ meats and oily fish. It is easily obtainable in capsule form from any health food store.

The story doesn't end there, though. Cholesterol is made in the liver through the mevalonate pathway. The HMG co-A reductase enzyme is the one responsible for initiating cholesterol. It is this enzyme which statins interfere with.

The same pathway is also responsible for the production of co-enzyme Q10. Q10 is an antioxidant combatting oxidative damage. It provides fuel for skeletal muscle and cardiac muscle. Without it we become weak and fatigued.

A further branch of the mevalonate pathway which is cut off by statins is the branch which produces nuclear factor kappa B (NF-KB). This disrupts the pathways which regulate the production of tau protein. Those living with Alzheimer's will be familiar with the concept of tau protein and its role in the progression of the disease.

In a nutshell, statins reduce cholesterol, co-enzyme Q10 and nuclear factor kappa B. The reduction or loss of these substances will negatively impact both body and brain.

Within this scenario of a disrupted mevalonate pathway we can see how a neurodegenerative process like MND can begin. What is troubling that we have forgotten what a healthy diet and lifestyle means. It has become a lifestyle choice to take statins in the erroneous belief that they will cause us no harm.

Steroids

Steroids are another medication which has some nasty side effects. While they are effective in reducing inflammation in the short term, they can induce a diabetic state and cause loss of muscle mass. The loss of muscle mass has not found to be reversible.

The Role of Antioxidants and Juicers in neuro-degenerative disorders (NDD's)

Fruit and vegetables and all their wonderful array of colours are full of antioxidants which are essential for calming neuro inflammatory processes. These are required in greater amounts for those with a NDD than those who do not have such a medical condition.

It can be difficult for those with a chronic medical condition to have the will or energy to prepare food which would help their condition, never mind have the appetite to cook it and eat it when all the preparation has been undertaken. It is at this point that a juicer becomes invaluable churning out jugs full of tasty blends of juice full of valuable antioxidants which are required by those with NDD's.

Everyone will have their own particular favourite make of juicer. Mine is the Matstone which produces glass after glass of the most flavoursome apple juice from our home grown apples. It leaves behind an almost dry fibre such is its ability to extract the goodness from the pulp.

Although our base juice is from apples, this is only because we have seven different varieties of apple tree which fruit prolifically from August onwards. To this base juice we can add carrots and broccoli, celery, blueberries – indeed anything that we have to hand that we fancy at the time. The choice is only limited by the imagination.

It is this beautiful cocktail of antioxidants that I believe should be prescribed for those with NDD's - not some unproven medication which may or may not prolong life by 2 months because nobody is quite sure what it does, if it does!

Two glasses full of this potent juice - and preferably three - should be considered part of the daily MND diet along with other potent – and proven - brain antioxidants mentioned in this book such as coffee and alpha lipoic acid. Olive oil contains many antioxidants so it can be sprinkled liberally over salads to increase the antioxidant potential in your diet.

Coffee as a powerful brain antioxidant

Coffee has been found to slow down the progression of motor neuron disease. It is packed with antioxidants and, as such, neutralises free radicals which are damaging to the brain.

Spices are powerful antioxidants and, as such have anti-inflammatory properties. They belong to a large group of bioactive compounds which are able to scavenge free radicals and form complexes with catalytic metal ions. This renders them inactive. Some catalytic ions such as iron are implicated in Parkinson's disease.

What does an MND diet look like?

The MND diet is a glorious one where butter cheese and eggs are allowed in quantity since it is not fat we are trying to limit. The only limitations placed on this diet are that omega 6 vegetable oils are eliminated and replaced with the stable saturated fats and further, that simple sugars are pared down as much as possible. A suitable substitute, for some,[26] is Hermeseta's liquid sweetener where a little goes a long way. It can be added to juices if they are too tart as well as, soups, beverages and baked products. It is very versatile. Contrary to belief, sweeteners aren't harmful and break down harmlessly to amino acids like phenylalanine, during digestion. The only contraindication may be for those with phenylketonuria.

In addition

- A juicer and soup maker are a must and a food processor will come in very handy.

---

[26] There is some concern that some individuals will not be able to tolerate artificial sweeteners for a number of reasons. In this case, the only option is to try and reduce the amount of sugar and processed foods as far as possible.

- Margarine is not recommended. At all times butter is far superior for brain health.
- A vitamin B complex tablet and vitamin D supplement, as outlined in earlier chapters, are recommended.
- Alpha lipoic acid (this in addition to the alpha-lipoic acid found in organ meats)
- Co-enzyme Q 10
- Whey protein - preferably 'free form' which is absorbed immediately as it requires no digesting.
- Two to three glass's full of mixed fruit and vegetable juice daily. Veer on the vegetable side as we are trying to keep the amount of fructose to the minimum while supplying antioxidants. This can be drunk as it is but whey protein can be added if a slightly thicker mix is required.
- Two helpings of organ meat weekly of approximately three ounce portions. This should only be reduced if an individual's iron levels are known to be on the high side in which case it is essential that alpha lipoic acid is taken in capsule form.
- Good quality protein at every meal (whey protein can be substituted at times).
- Good quality protein sources include fish, meat, milk, cheese, eggs, yogurt and nuts.
- At least two cups of good quality strong coffee daily.
- Use olive oil, wheat germ oil and nut oils liberally. Most of these oils burn at very low temperatures. A

spoonful of wheat germ oil or wheat germ itself can be sprinkled into soups, on porridge. The idea is to increase the number of antioxidants in the diet and these oils provide plenty of vitamin E which is essential for brain health. Keep all oils stored in the refrigerator and away from light.
- Sauté vegetables in butter gently or add butter after steaming
- Add a knob of butter to soups
- Juice a number of vegetables and use this as a base for soup
- Use olive oil liberally on salads and vegetable dishes
- Add coffee to sponge mix
- Sprinkle wheat germ on cereals to enhance vitamin E intake
- Add spices such as cinnamon, nutmeg to dishes
- Use turmeric often as it has anti-inflammatory properties. Those countries who use it a lot in their cooking have been found to have lower rates of NDD's.

Why use a juicer?

The concept of having five a day – or even ten a day – helpings of fruit and vegetables, becomes less daunting with the use of a juicer, even in the hands of the most reluctant cook or those with very poor appetites. A good juicer will simply extract all the juice and leave the pulp behind. When I have used the Matstone, the pulp is just about dry it is so good at what it does.

Just drinking the high antioxidant juice can be beneficial. Many people with NDD's have impaired gut motility and adding more and more fibre is not to be recommended and can cause a great deal of discomfort as well as loss of appetite. Sorbitol, a sugar found in fruit – aids gut motility and is present in the juice. However, the recommendation is that the juice comes from mainly vegetable sources if this is not too unpalatable.

Latest Research

The copper connection

Superoxide dismutase (SOD) is an enzyme that helps break down potentially harmful oxygen molecules. These molecules have the potential to damage tissues including neuronal tissue.

The SOD protein requires copper to function and this is delivered to the SOD protein by a copper chaperone.

Sometimes a mutant form of SOD is present. It has 'gain of function.' This means that through its mutation it gains a new function which is almost always dominant in its expression. The copper chaperone for SOD completes the maturation for SOD but the copper chaperone inadvertently causes the demise of mice, through deterioration and death of motor neurons, within two weeks of birth when involved in the maturation and expression of mutant SOD.

Mitochondria – which are the powerhouses of energy in a cell – require copper as a cofactor for the two enzymes that they contain. A copper deficiency affects mitochondria during their development that is consistent with a copper deficiency seen in the spinal cords of ALS patients.

A copper ligand CuATSM - used in PET imaging - has been found to extend life in high expressing mutant SOD (SOD$^{G93A)}$ mice by up to 25%. It has been found that MND can be restarted and stopped by constantly stopping and starting the treatment.

The delivery of the copper ligand to spinal cords has been undertaken using DMSO – an easily obtainable solvent as CuATSM easily dissolves in it. It is then applied to the spinal cord. It is able to cross the blood brain barrier.

While this research is still ongoing, it does show the importance of copper and that a simple copper deficiency can impact neural health negatively. As excessive copper is just as problematical as a deficiency then it is recommended that copper supplementation is not undertaken unless on medical advice. Good sources of copper are beef liver and dark chocolate.

Copper kills bacteria, viruses and fungi on contact so maintaining optimum levels will reduce the risk of infection.

Protective and risk factors for ALS

A study looked at specific foods to verify if nutrients could be risk factors or protective factors for amyotrophic lateral sclerosis (ALS).

The study comprised of 212 cases of those newly diagnosed with ALS and 212 controls.

The results are tabulated below:

Foods associated with risk reduction	Foods associated with risk increase
Coffee and tea	Red meat
Wholemeal bread	Pork and processed meat
Raw vegetables	Total protein (OR 2.96)
Citrus fruits (contain flavonoids)	Animal protein (OR 2.91)
	Sodium (OR[27] 3.96)
	Zinc* (OR 2.78)
	Glutamic acid (3.63)

The conclusions drawn were that some food have a protective factor for ALS and other foods are a risk factor.

It should be noted that a risk factor is not a causative factor.

---

[27] An odds ratio (OR) is a measure of association between and exposure and outcome. ... the *p* value, the 95% CI does not report a measure's statistical significance.

*Zinc is required to activate T regulatory cells and it is this increase in Tregs that we desire if we are to slow the progression of microglia and the advance of MND. It may be that the increased availability of zinc reflects the body's requirement for this trace mineral. Further, zinc is a powerful antiviral and any infective agent that is potentially contributing to the disease process will be effectively weakened by optimum amounts of zinc.

Similarly, glutamic acid is required to neutralise ammonia that is formed when cells are broken down during injury and infection. The presence of increased serum glutamic acid levels may also indicate the body's 'recognition' that it needs to increase glutamic acid in a protective role rather than as indicating a risk factor.

Flavonoids have antioxidant activity and have the ability to reduce free radical formation and to scavenge free radicals. Coffee, tea, raw vegetables, citrus fruits

Heating is accountable for the oxidation, thermal degradation and leaching of bioactive compounds from fresh vegetables.[28] This explains why raw vegetables have a protective factor for ALS as opposed to cooked vegetables. However, this is not as clear cut as it appears. Some fruits and vegetables along with their antioxidants are absorbed better when cooked. One such antioxidant is lycopene which gives tomatoes its red colour.

28

https://www.sciencedirect.com/science/article/pii/S1021949814001379#bib2

In addition, raw fruit and vegetables contain enzymes. Enzymes speed up metabolic reactions that are necessary for the health of the body but enzymes are easily destroyed by heat. It follows that a diet of fresh fruit and raw vegetables are important for health.

A study[29] showed that wheat, one of the most important grains in the world, is not only a source of basic nutrients, such as carbohydrates, proteins, and vitamins, but also a source of antioxidants, such as flavonoids and phenolic acids. It was reported that the antioxidant activity of whole grain including whole wheat bread ranged from 1303 to 2479 µmol trolox*** equivalent (TE) per 100 g, whereas the average values of 24 types of fruit and 22 types of vegetables were 2200 and 1200 µmol TE per 100 g, respectively. These results indicated that whole grains have pronounced antioxidant activities that should not be overlooked.

---

[29] https://www.sciencedirect.com/science/article/pii/S2214514115000471
***A trolox is basically the strength of antioxidant activity

Recipes

Soup Recipes (all of the ingredients can be adjusted to taste and some ingredients omitted and others added, for this reason, quantities are not given since individual tastes differ).

Non flavoured whey protein can be sprinkled over any of the soup to add extra protein.

A teaspoon of turmeric can be added to soups if it is unlikely to detract from the flavour. It is all about personal choice.

Soups can be batch made and frozen (apart from Drop Egg Soup which does not freeze well although the first stage chicken stock can be made beforehand and frozen for later use)

Sometimes if the taste of the soup isn't quite balanced then I add a

- Few drops of Hermesetas sweetener
- Herbs and spices
- Dollop of yogurt
- Lemon juice.
- Apple juice or other fruit juices

Chicken and Pineapple Soup

Ingredients

One apple chopped
Onion
Chopped chicken
Pineapple chunks in juice or fresh pineapple (save the juice to add to the mix)
Celery
Garlic
Seasoning
Chilli flakes

Butter added once the soup is cooked.

Whey protein or skimmed milk powder can always be whizzed in at the end for extra protein.

Method
Place all the ingredients in the soup maker and add the pineapple juice, top up with water to the levels required by the soup maker.
Set the mode – smooth or chunky.
Once cooked, add a knob of butter.

Basil and Tomato Soup

Ingredients

Tin of chopped tomatoes or fresh plum tomatoes
Bunch of basil
Chopped onions
Garlic
Seasoning
Knob of butter to be added after the soup has cooked and/or yogurt.
Parmesan cheese or other if desired.

Method

Place the first five ingredients in the soup maker and top up to level with water.
Set the mode.
When cooked add a knob of butter and sprinkle with cheese.

Lentil and Vegetable Soup.

Ingredients

Lentils soaked overnight and then cooked in the soup maker before adding other ingredients,

Onion
Garlic
Mixed vegetables

One apple chopped
Seasoning
Knob of butter
Grated cheese

Method

Add the first five ingredients to the lentil 'soup' and add water to the correct level in the soup maker.
Set the mode
Once cooked add a knob of butter

Pea Soup

Ingredients

Frozen peas

Chopped onion

Garlic

Celery

Potato

Seasoning

Knob of butter

Skimmed milk powder

Method

Place the first six ingredients in the soup maker and add water to the recommended level.

Set the mode.

Once cooked add skimmed milk powder and the knob of butter and whizz for about ten seconds.

Leek and potato

Ingredients

Leek

Potato

Garlic

Onion

Seasoning

Knob of butter

Skimmed milk powder

Method

Add the first five ingredients to the soup maker and add water to the correct level.

Set the mode.

Once cooked add the knob of butter and skimmed milk powder and whizz for around ten seconds.

Drop Egg Soup – two stages. (The first stage is not for the soup maker – this needs a non-stick saucepan)

Ingredients

Proper home- made chicken stock (see below)

Pak choir (finely chopped)

Onion (finely chopped)

Garlic

Chinese Five Spice

Red pepper (finely chopped)

Celery (finely chopped)

Sweetcorn

Seasoning

Eggs

Method

Place the chicken stock in a non- stick pan with finely diced onion, celery, garlic, seasoning, pepper, Five Spice and sweetcorn. Cook gently for about five minutes. Add some of the pack choir.

Barely whisk the eggs. Take the soup off the heat. Drizzle the eggs into the soup barely stirring as you do so. Immediately this is done, serve.

Once in serving dishes throw the remaining Pak Choi over the soup.

Chicken stock (a slow cooker is useful for this).

Place the carcase of a chicken in water and cover. Add about one tablespoon of vinegar or lemon juice.

Slowly simmer until the bones are dropping apart. Separate the stock from the bones. Throw the bones away.

- Please note that chicken is pro-inflammatory hence why chicken soup is known as Jewish penicillin since it helps gear the immune system into action at times of illness. It is at times of illness that it can be taken. It should not be discounted entirely as it contains lots of healthy amino acids such as glucosamine which have been found to aid joint health. Wisdom will dictate its use.

Pork and Apricot Soup

Ingredients

Pork tenderloin

Tinned or fresh apricots

Onion

Garlic

Seasoning

Potato chopped small

Method

Place all the ingredients in the soup maker and add water to the recommended level.

Set the mode (I normally set it on chunky but puree it for about ten seconds at the end)

When cooked add a knob of butter.

The ultimate nerve regenerating soup

I have given it this name as it contains a high number of ingredients which have been proven to regenerate nerve endings as they contain butyric acid. The ingredients are the lentils, beans, butter and parmesan cheese.

Lentils also contain tryptophan which is an amino acid that is the precursor to serotonin a substance which has anti- anxiety properties. I once made some of my lentil soup with home-made chicken stock to a guest. He liked it so much that he had two large bowls full whereupon he promptly fell asleep and did not wake up until some hours later. I always recommend lentils to anyone who has trouble sleeping or is beset by anxiety.

Ingredients

Lentils soaked overnight and then cooked well in the soup maker or non-stick pan, before adding other ingredients.

One apple
Onion
Garlic
Seasoning
Selection of cooked beans – kidney, aduki, haricot, chick peas etc. as these have nerve regenerating properties. Some supermarkets sell tins of ready cooked mixed beans which can be used. Rinse them well as we are trying to reduce the amount of salt eaten.

Knob of butter - has nerve regenerating properties
Grated cheese (preferably parmesan as this has the most nerve regenerating properties)
Skimmed milk powder

Method
Add ingredients 1-4 to the cook lentil stock in the pan or soup maker and cook.
Set the mode if using the soup maker.
Add the cooked beans towards the end of the cooking to heat through.
Whizz in a knob of butter and skimmed milk powder.
Sprinkle grated cheese over once served.

Puddings

Chocolate or coffee steamed sponge with chocolate or coffee sauce. (full of antioxidants)

Ingredients (for four people)

6 ounces of flour (preferably whole wheat although this gives a chewier texture) or replace some with ground nuts eg ground almonds
3 eggs beaten
4 ounces of butter
2 ounces of sugar
Hermesetas liquid sweetener or similar

Two tablespoons of cocoa powder (NOT drinking chocolate) or two tablespoons of coffee granules approximately.

Method

Mix the first five ingredients together then depending on whether you want a coffee or chocolate steamed sponge
Add either half of the above of the cocoa powder as it is, or
Half the coffee diluted in a small amount of warm water. Mix well.

Place in pudding bowl and steam until cooked OR this could be placed in a microwave for approximately 5-6 minutes for speed although it isn't quite as soft.

Chocolate or Coffee sauce

Heat some milk in a saucepan
Combine cocoa powder with some cornflour and mix with a little cold water, if making chocolate sauce or
Add coffee granules directly to the milk. Mix the cornflour to cold water separately.

Add sweetener to taste.

When the milk is nearly boiling stir in the cornflour mix and stir well until the sauce thickens.

Variation

Add chopped walnuts to the pudding or sauce to add vitamin E, omega 3's and extra calories.

Nut crumble to top fruit

Ingredients

6 ounces of mixed plain flour and chopped nuts
3 ounces of butter
1   ounce of sugar
 Pinch of spice (generally nutmeg or cinnamon)

Fruit of choice
Hermesetas to sweeten fruit, if desired

Method
Mix first four ingredients together to make a crumbly nut mix.

Place fruit in bottom of a pie dish and sweeten with sweetener if required.

Cover with nut crumble and bake until golden at no higher than 180C.

This dish freezes well.

Variation
Dot the crumble with a little butter and sprinkle with a mix of brown sugar and cinnamon.

Serve with yogurt as fermented foods add vitamin K to the diet which does impact positively on brain health, too.

Egg Custard

Ingredients

Half a pint of full fat milk
Two or three eggs
Vanilla essence to taste
Sweetener
 Pinch of nutmeg
Knob of butter

Method

Simply mix all the ingredients together well. Don't worry the nutmeg will rise to the top of the mixture. Tip into a baking dish. Cook on a very low heat until just about set. There will always be a little runniness due to the whey from the milk.

Apple Loaf (eat sliced and spread with butter)

Pureed apple is a good substitute for eggs in cakes and puddings or use both. In this recipe I'll keep the apple in since it needs to reflect its name. I'll leave it up to you whether you want to keep the eggs in but taking them out will reduce many important nutrients necessary for brain health.

Ingredients
6 ounces of self-raising flour and one tsp of bicarbonate of soda.
Four ounces of butter
Two eggs lightly beaten
2   tablespoon of whey protein
Cup of pureed apple
Teaspoon of mixed spice
Two ounces of sugar
Cup of mixed dried fruit left to soak in strong tea for one hour. Chopped dates are good in a cake like this but sultanas and raisins are also favourites.
Ground nuts if desired

Method.
Drain mixed fruit well. Add to all the other ingredients. Mix well. Add a little milk if the mix is too dry.

Oven method - Line a loaf tin and drop mixture in smoothing the top out. Sprinkle with a little brown sugar if desired. Bake at 180C for 30-40 minutes until mixture springs back

Microwave method - mix all ingredients as above. Place in microwaveable loaf mould.
Microwave for approximately six minutes. If it doesn't spring back at this stage add 30 seconds more and test again until you have the desired result

Leave to cool. Slice and wrap in greaseproof paper before freezing.

Chocolate beetroot cake

Ingredients
8 oz self-raising flour or 4 oz of flour and 4oz of ground almonds
3 eggs beaten
6 oz of butter
4oz fresh beetroot grated
3 tbls cocoa powder
2- 3 oz sugar/ Hermesetas drops if further sweetener is needed
Milk to mix
1 tsp bicarbonate of soda

Method
Cream the butter and sugar together.

Add a little of the flour, eggs, cocoa powder and bicarbonate of soda to the mixture at a time.
When mixed in fold in the beetroot well.
Add sweetener to taste.
Add milk until a dropping consistency is reached or flour if the mixture is too wet.

Place in an 8" cake tin and bake at 180C for 25 minutes. Test to see if it is springy. If not place back in the oven and bake further testing every 10 minutes or so for springiness. If the cake looks as though it is browning too quickly then cover the top with foil.

The cake can also be microwaved in a microwave safe mould for six minutes. Leave for a minute then test for springiness before deciding whether to microwave for another minute.

The cake can be spread with melted dark chocolate.
A filling of butter softened with melted chocolate, sweetener and ground almonds will add to necessary nutrients for brain health. Cream cheese can be substituted for the butter, if desired.

Ice cream and sauces for Ice cream

Banana Ice cream and variations on a theme

Mash two bananas well with some cream or yogurt and sweetener if desired. Freeze for at least an hour

Stew any fruit until all juice has reduced well. Take some Greek yogurt or similar and mix with a tablespoon or so of whey protein. Add sweetener to the fruit and cream mix and slowly drag the fruit through the whey mix in a swirl. Freeze for at least an hour before eating.
Most sauces for ice-cream are heavily sugared. As sugar causes neuro-inflammation we need to avoid this at all costs.

Whey protein can be added to dilute strong coffee or cocoa with sweetener if desired to produce a passable sauce. It needs a good whisk as whey protein does not mix easily but it can be done. Ground almond blended with the cocoa powder is a nice touch just as pieces of walnut added to the coffee sauce is.

Rum and raisin
Other flavours which you could add to whey protein are a little rum flavouring or real rum if you prefer, in which some raisins have soaked in. Take these to one side and only add them when you have your rum sauce ready. You may need to add sweetener

Orange sauce – use good quality orange juice either homemade or shop bought and whisk well with the whey, add sweetener as desired. If you have some pieces of chopped orange segments to add to the sauce, the better. Treat other citrus fruits in the same way.

Lime sauce
To the basic lime sauce (see how the orange sauce is made above) add coconut or very dark chocolate bits. Don't forget the sweetener.

Off course any fruit can be slowly stewed until it forms a sauce or coulis. The addition of sweetener may be required for some of the tarter fruits

Fruit ice lollies

Press some juice from apples or other fruit. Place in a plastic cup with a lolly stick and freeze.

Variations

- Apple and carrot juice
- Combination of forest fruits stewed slowly and put through a jelly bag. Use the liquid for ice lollies and use the pulp over ice cream, added to other fruit in a crumble or to a cake mix.

Some brain healthy mains, starters and, accompaniments.

Curry

Curry is a great way to take in lots of antioxidants provided by the spices. Everybody, if they like curry, has their favourite dish and combination of spices. I use home- made meat stock in mine.

The yellow spice in curry – turmeric – contains very small amounts of curcumin. This substance reduces oxidised LDL cholesterol and protects artery walls from the effects of homocysteine. Homocysteine is an amino acid by product which can damage blood vessel walls.

Ingredients

Diced meat of choice
Onions
Garlic
Sultanas or apricots if desired – the latter chopped finely
Jar of curry paste
Home- made meat stock
Tomatoes quartered
Peppers if desired
Any other vegetables you might like

Method

Cook the chicken in a little oil with the onions and garlic and choice of vegetables

Add the curry paste and cook according to instructions adding chicken stock as required

Ten minutes before the recommended time add the fruit – sultanas and apricot etc., to taste.

Serve with a preferred accompaniment. I find that rice cooks very well in the microwave. Scoop out enough for your needs, Cover with boiling water. Cook in the microwave for ten minutes.

Brown rice takes a little longer so I cook it for twenty minutes in the microwave and then leave it for ten minutes to absorb the water. I add more boiling water as required and then cook in the microwave for another ten minutes.

To raise the antioxidant level, you could add half a teaspoon of cinnamon or a cinnamon stick. Stir with a knob of butter at the end or add it to the curry to raise butyric acid levels.

Cauliflower Rice – this is a good substitute for rice if you need to increase the amount of choline in the diet.

Offal Shepherd's Pie
When my children were little and cash was hard to come by, I was fortunate that liver was a cheap meal and, even better, my children did not object to it. However, I did not

want to serve it up as slices every time. One day I minced it up, added onions and fried it before topping with mashed potato. I used lamb's liver as the flavour is fairly mild compared to beef or pig's liver. The children did not notice that it was not the usual beef mince and pronounced it an excellent shepherd's pie.

If the potato is mashed with plenty of butter and some lentils are added to the minced liver, then more butyric acid is added. Sprinkle grated cheese over the potato and you have added even more butyric acid – the substance which regenerates nerve endings. The minced liver provides plenty of the antioxidant, alpha lipoic acid and a building block of protein, glutamic acid. Vitamin D is stored in the liver and so there are good amounts of this fat soluble vitamin in liver. The vitamin in greatest amounts to be found in liver is vitamin A and current recommendations are that pregnant women should not eat more than two helpings of liver weekly.

I am not against adding a teaspoon of pure cocoa powder to the meat. This may sound strange but without the addition of sugar, cocoa has little, if any discernible flavour. All it does in a dish of this sort is add valuable antioxidants.

Gravy

I am not in favour of the very salty cubes that can be bought at the supermarket. Salt is a risk factor for MND. In the winter – when the Aga is on - I dry and grind my own vegetables and herbs and make my own dried stock. It generally lasts the whole year round but now and again I like a change. If I have some woody bits of celery or turnip or apple core etc. then I will put them through the Matstone and extract the juice. I will save up bits of inedible veg in the freezer for such a time as this. Heated up the vegetable juice, thickened with a little cornflour makes a delicate gravy for a Shepherd's pie.

On other occasions, if I do not have any spare inedible vegetables I will dice a mix I take from the garden, although frozen will do, and make a vegetable gravy in the soup maker. If half an apple is added to the mix it generally does not need thickening since the apple provides plenty of pectin which thickens the gravy.

I always add onions – not just because I like them but because they contain quercetin which is another anti-inflammatory antioxidant.

I will render bones from any meat source down in the slow cooker, adding any spare vegetables which I have. The beauty of bone broth is that it contains glycine, a small amino acid which is vital for the health of connective tissue. Gelatine is made from glycine (as are gummy bears and jelly……… and that wonderful jelly found in pork pies) and often NDD's do not arrive in isolation. They are often accompanied by other inflammatory conditions.

Vegetarian Cheese and Tomato Bake (serves 4-6)

Ingredients

Two tins of chopped tomatoes
One tablespoon of tomato paste
Mustard and pepper for the cheese sauce
Grated cheese – leave some aside for the top of the bake
Knob of butter
Cooked pasta
A pint of homemade cheese sauce (one pint of milk heated, thicken with cornflour mixed in a little cold water first, take off the heat and add grated cheese, seasoning and mustard)

Method
Mix all together well in a baking dish. Sprinkle the left over grated cheese over the bake.
Place in the oven at 180C until nicely browned.

This dish freezes well and can be cut up into squares as individual portions.

Filled bell pepper (vegetarian)

Ingredients
Bell peppers cut in half and seeds taken out
Vegetable spaghetti, lightly steamed
Cheese sauce
Grated cheese
Breadcrumbs
Knob of butter
Pepper

Method
Place vegetable spaghetti in the bell pepper
Pour cheese sauce over the spaghetti
Sprinkle top with pepper, breadcrumbs and grated cheese. Add a knob of butter.

Bake for 10-15 minutes in an oven heated to 180C or grill until browned to taste, as preferred.

Dictionary of Terms

ALA – alpha lipoic acid – inhibits inappropriate microglial activation.

Arginine – an amino acid that neutralises ammonia and is beneficial for neurodegenerative disorders.

Astrocytes – these are neuroglia like microglia. They are distributed in non-overlapping regions in the CNS.

Cysteine – *chemi*cal formula HS CH_2 CH (NH_2) COOH is a sulphur containing amino acid

GABA – gamma amino butyric acid – an inhibitory amino acid which relieves anxiety and pain. Its precursor is glutamic acid.

Glutamate is a powerful excitatory neurotransmitter that is released by neurons in the brain. It is responsible for transmitting messages between nerve cells. It plays a role in learning and memory.

Glutamic Acid - the brain's primary food and used in the synthesis of glutamine and GABA. Its use is the only way that the brain detoxifies itself by removing toxic ammonia from neurons. Glutamic acid also boosts glutathione which is a powerful antioxidant. It provides a direct energy source to the brain which increases mental alertness and memory function.

Glutamine – an amino acid which is found stored in muscles and is also a by- product of glutamic acid and toxic ammonia ie glutamic acid neutralises toxic ammonia producing harmless glutamine in the process.

Glycine – the smallest amino acid – a deficiency is implicated in many disease states. Glycine infusion has been found to prevent microglial activation which is implicated in the progression of MND. Glycine can also reverse type 2 diabetes. Studies[30] have also shown that autistic spectrum disorder is a manifestation of systemic glycine deficiency It occurs as a result of the consumption of a typical diet high in essential amino acids but lacking in glycine.

There is a critical threshold concentration of plasma glycine that must be maintained for the overall optimal regulation of the innate immune system to which microglia belong.

Homocysteine – an amino acid by product – found in the methionine cycle - which can damage the linings of blood vessels if not converted back to methionine quickly. In order for this to be achieved, it needs vitamins B3, B6 and folic acid. It has the chemical formula

$HS\ CH_2\ CH_2\ CH\ (NH_2)\ COOH$

Inflammation plays a role in MND disease progression. Non neuronal cells like microglia or astrocytes are activated during other immune cells such as monocytes and natural killer cells which cross the blood brain barrier. When microglia are activated they release various substances known to be toxic to neurons. These include oxygen radicals, glutamate and nitric oxide.

---

[30] https://www.bmj.com/content/361/bmj.k1674/rr-3

Lecithin - means 'egg yolk.' The best sources of phospholipids are found in wheat germ, peanuts, cauliflower, grape juice and liver. They are a mood enhancer and protect against memory decline. The neurotransmitter acetylcholine is built from choline derived from phosphatidyl choline.

Leucine – this is an amino acid which is used by the liver, fat tissue and muscle tissue, mainly. Leucine is currently suspected to be the only amino acid which can stimulate muscle growth as well as preventing deterioration of muscle with age. It is mainly found in cheese, soybeans, beef, chicken, pork, nuts, seeds, fish, seafood and beans. The requirements for any individual is approximately 17.7mg for every pound of body weight. It also slows the passage of pain signals to the CNS.

Mevalonate Pathway - an important metabolic pathway which has numerous branches involved in the synthesis of important products such as cholesterol, isoprenoids (vital for diverse cellular functions) and Coenzyme Q10 amongst others.

Microglia - they are a type of neuroglia located throughout the brain and spinal cord. They comprise 10-15% of the cells in the brain and they are the main form of the active immune defence in the brain.
Microglia present antigen in the brain. This is a 3 step process
1. Engagement of the Major Histocompatibility Complex with regulatory T cells (TCr)
2. The binding of stimulating molecules

3. Secretion or expression of T cell polarising molecules in specific population of Antigen Presenting Cells.

(Note the dendritic cells are the main APC in the peripheral immune system but may participate in the regulation of T cell responses within the CNS.)

Microglia constantly scavenge for plaques and molecular junk, synapses and infectious agents. They are extremely sensitive to small pathological changes in the CNS. This sensitivity is achieved, partly, through the presence of potassium channels as they will respond to minute changes in extracellular potassium.

The action of microglia can be understood better when the function of the blood brain barrier is considered. The blood brain barrier's job is to prevent pathogens from invading the CNS. However, if pathogens do cross, antibodies are not available from the body to deal with them. The microglia then act as APC's and activate T cells which protect cells and repair injuries in the CNS.

Methionine – an essential amino acid, found in casein and egg white with the chemical formula $CH_3 S\ CH_2\ CH_2\ CH\ (NH_2)\ COOH$

Oxygen radicals – when oxygen atoms separate they have an unpaired electron. Electrons like to be in pairs so, as they are highly reactive, they take electrons off DNA, proteins and cells, damaging them in the process. In the brain, the microglia will become activated when any damage occurs and signal to other cells in the immune system. In addition, they initiate a 'mopping up' process.

Phenylalanine – an amino acid that curbs hunger. It is a major part of collagen and treats MND diseases and disorders.

Phosphatidyl choline is comprised of B vitamins, choline, phosphoric acid, gamma linoleic acid, and inositol. It is also the key building block of the cell membrane and a protector from cell oxidation.

Quercetin – an antioxidant of flavonol pigment in the form of glycosides with chemical formula $C_{15} H_5 O_2 (OH)$

Riluzole – an unproven medication which reduces the amount of glutamic acid in the brain thus

- depriving the brain of its ability to detoxify itself
- Depriving the brain of its direct energy source and thus decreasing mental alertness and memory function
- Depriving the brain of its means to make GABA, an inhibitory neurotransmitter, that reduces anxiety and pain
- Inhibiting the restoration of brain function after injury.
- Preventing the upregulation of Tregs which are necessary for slowing down the progression of MND. (Glutamic acid increases the upregulation of Tregs).

Riluzole was the first FDA approved medication for amyotrophic lateral sclerosis. It was approved for ALS because in several clinical trials it modestly extended survival or time for insertion of a feeding tube. Initial clinical trial reports of a slowing of muscle deteriorations or symptomatic benefits were not corroborated in subsequent studies [31]

---

[31]Bensimon et al 1994 Lancomblez 1996

Pharmacoeconomics research has challenged the cost-effectiveness of Riluzole treatment of ALS [32]

Adverse events include blurred vision, difficulty breathing, weakness, dizziness, gastrointestinal discomfort among others.

Concerns Over Riluzole

Riluzole's mechanism of action is not fully understood. It has, in studies shown repeatedly to modulate glutamate neurotransmission by inhibiting both glutamate release and post synaptic glutamate receptor signalling. It has been reported to be neuroprotective by suppressing astrocytosis [33]

Riluzole has been shown to inhibit the release of glutamic acid from cultured neurons, from brain slices and from corticostriatal neurons in vivo. However, while it may do this, it has still not been demonstrated that there is any association between excessive glutamic acid and motor neuron disease. In fact, the link between hyper excitability and disease still has to be established.

In light of findings that repeatedly show that Riluzole does not impact the course of the disease and further, induces some nasty side effects, it is unclear why it continues to be prescribed.

Further, a perfectly harmless non-proteinaceous amino acid, L-theanine – found mainly in green and black tea acts as a glutamate antagonist. This means that it blocks the action of

---

[32] Messori et al 1999
[33] Martin etl al 1993, Hubert et al 1994, Carbone et al 2012

glutamate which is a neurotransmitter found in the brain that is implicated in the progression of MND.

L-theanine is neuroprotective.[34] It is the substance which provides the feeling of calm and 'all is well with the world' that you feel when you have a drink of tea. It has no known negative side effects.

In contrast to the unproven effects of Riluzole, research has found an association between coffee intake and slower progression of MND, in that the greater the intake of coffee, the slower the progression of the disease.

The chemical composition of coffee and what it has to offer in the treatment of MND seems to be a far worthier candidate for research. Further, it does not carry the multiplicity of side effects that can be found with Riluzole, which has the potential to impact on the quality of life for those with MND.

Serine – an amino acid from which part of the myelin sheath – which covers and protects nerve fibres - is formed.

Super Dismutase (SOD) is a metabolic enzyme. It has antioxidant properties that assist in the neutralising of the free radical superoxide which is highly destructive to cells.

Taurine – this amino acid aids the cleansing of free radical waste.

Theanine (L-theanine)

---

[34] https://www.ncbi.nlm.nih.gov/pubmed/23097345

A non proteinaceous amino acid that is mainly found in green and black tea which blocks glutamate receptors thus promoting a feeling of calm and relaxation. It is also a precursor to GABA which is the major inhibitory neurotransmitter.

Research around the protective effects of coffee and antioxidants

Antioxidants

These are substances that can prevent or slow down damage to cells caused by free radicals.

Free radicals, also known as reactive oxygen species, are unstable molecules that are produced by the body. They are the result of processes that the body undergoes, such as inflammation, or as a result of environmental stress in the form of cigarette smoke, sun exposure or pollution such as car exhaust fumes. If the free radicals cannot be removed quickly enough then oxidative damage occurs. Oxidative damage is linked to a large number of diverse diseases that include:

- Motor neuron disease
- Parkinson's disease
- Respiratory disease
- Cancer

- Arthritis
- Stroke
- Any chronic inflammatory disease

Antioxidants are sometimes called 'free radical scavengers.' They help to neutralise free radicals in our body. The body makes some of its own antioxidants but many antioxidants come from plants. The body, however, cannot make its own antioxidants without the ingestion of correct nutritional substances.

Most of these substances are found in fresh fruit and vegetables. Vitamin C, however, although a superb antioxidant, is easily destroyed by sunlight; it dissipates rapidly the longer it is stored.

Different foods provide different antioxidants. A diverse diet is necessary to avoid disease states that often appear to be instigated by a healthy lifestyle. For example, excessive exercise, in itself may lead to oxidative stress with the capacity to induce serious injury. However, if this exercise also results in tissue trauma then the level of free radicals rises rapidly with even further potential to cause serious illness especially if the activity is undertaken in polluted surroundings.

Some other activities and processes that increase the number of free radicals are:

- Sugary and refined foods consumption, trans fats
- Radiation
- Exposure to pesticides, chemicals, drugs and chemotherapy

- Industrial solvents
- Normal mitochondrial function

A study[35] argued that the human body is in a constant battle to keep from aging. Research[36] suggests that free radical damage to cells leads to the pathological changes associated with ageing.

Studies[37] have shown that coffee drinkers are less likely to get ALS, Parkinson's disease and Alzheimer's disease. These are all diseases of advancing age. In a study[3] of elderly mice with Alzheimer's disease, for example, caffeine was found to reverse cognitive impairment as well as lowering brain amyloid-beta levels.

In an animal model of ALS, coffee was found to increase antioxidant enzyme capacity in the brain of male G39A mice, improving motor performance.

A caffeine derivative, known as LM11A-24 appears to protect degenerating motor neurons.[38]

---

[35] https://www.ncbi.nlm.nih.gov/pmc/articles/PMC3249911/

[36] Ashok BT, Ali R. The aging paradox: Free radical theory of aging. Exp Gerontol. 1999;34:293–303.

[37] https://academic.oup.com/aje/article/174/9/1002/168671
[38] https://www.ncbi.nlm.nih.gov/pubmed/17004921

This is all well and good but coffee, whether decaffeinated, or not, has been found to slow down the progression of MND.

Coffee contains a number of important antioxidants as well as vitamin B3. Niacin is added to – and found in- a great many foods so it is less likely that this is the important nutrient that slows the progression of MND.

Science Direct[39] states that:

Coffee beans are a rich source of biologically active compounds such as caffeine, chlorogenic acids, nicotinic acid, trigonelline, cafestol, and kahweol, which have significant potential as antioxidants.

It is worth exploring these antioxidants a little further.

Chlorogenic acids

These have a wide array of benefits including having an anti-inflammatory effect in the brain.

---

[39] https://www.sciencedirect.com/science/article/pii/B9780124047389000039

Trigonelline –

This substance has many potential benefits.[40] It is neuroprotective, anti-migraine and reduces neuron excitability.

Cafestol and kahweol

Both of these substances tend to impact positively on the liver lowering inflammation in this organ. While there do not appear to be, at the moment, any studies linking liver disease with MND, there are studies[41] that link liver and gut activity with Alzheimer's disease. The brain is intricately connected to all other organs.

---

[40] https://www.researchgate.net/publication/225288518_Trigonelline_A_Plant_Alkaloid_with_Therapeutic_Potential_for_Diabetes_and_Central_Nervous_System_Disease

[41] https://www.alzheimersresearchuk.org/new-findings-link-activity-gut-liver-alzheimers-risk/

Thank you for purchasing this book. Every time a book is purchased, a donation is made to one of the charities I am currently supporting. These can be found on my author's website. See below.

Other Health Related Books by the Author

- **The Reluctant Bowel**
- **A Weighty Issue**
- **Sleep, Perchance to Dream**
- **The Journey: EDS and chronic pain**
- **The MND diet: using nutrition to slow down the progress of neurodegeneration**
- **A Necessary Sorrow**
- **Treat infection Naturally**
- **Successful Aging**
- **Taking another Road: Pain: its causes and what can be done about it**
- **Osteoarthritis and Pain**
- **A Treatment Strategy for Migraine**

These can be found here on the author's page

https://www.amazon.co.uk/-/e/B07BPQZ5CD

You may also be interested in the semi-autobiographical trilogy of the authors life found in these three books

- The Prejudged
- Where the Blackbird Never Sings
- A Summer's Symphony

And the author's children's books

- Fanny and Victorian Jack
- Fanny and the Gamekeeper's Cottage

If you have found this book useful, I would be grateful if you would leave a review.

This book will be updated in line with new research regularly. Thank you!

Printed in Great
Britain
by Amazon